THE BOOK
OF FLOATING

The aim of CONSCIOUSNESS CLASSICS is to bring to life significant publications in the consciousness field, which have not been available, and to showcase new books which are destined to become classics.

CONSCIOUSNESS CLASSICS conserves these texts as the authors originally intended them, in a carefully re-designed contemporary format for new generations of readers. These books are an important legacy of groundbreaking consciousness explorers of the 20th century.

MICHAEL HUTCHISON

THE BOOK
OF FLOATING

EXPLORING THE PRIVATE SEA

GATEWAYS BOOKS AND TAPES
NEVADA CITY, CALIFORNIA

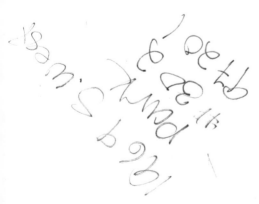

CONTENTS

FOREWORD

I thought Michael was great before I ever met him. He wrote an article in a well respected, internationally circulated New York newspaper *The Village Voice* that doubled the traffic in my Beverly Hills Tank Center, and what he wrote didn't offend me or misrepresent any of the things I believed to be true. Moreover his writing style was engaging, intelligent, bright and shiny. The people who came to use the floatation tanks as a result of reading his article were filled with information and expectations of a variety of good things happening—and they did happen.

When I actually met Michael Hutchison in New Orleans at the Second International Conference on REST and Self-Regulation—the gathering of scientists, researchers and entrepreneurs focused on the promise of the tank—I thought that the floatation tank now had a valuable ally. Michael seemed interesting and interested, original, and an excellent, well-researched writer. We collaborated for many years whenever we had the chance. The biggest project was the first West Coast "MegaBrain" workshop filling our Los Angeles factory with thousands of eager folks sampling the newest mind machines that were just being introduced to a receptive audience.

I didn't see him much for many years but I was hearing about him a lot since he was now a celebrity speaking at all the Consciousness Conferences, giving workshops, and recognized as one of the leading authorities in the field. He actually mid-wived—"MegaBrain". Michael was a public hero—a pied piper of life improvement.

And then he vanished—disappeared. I heard rumors—all of them bad. I heard stories of such a long run of bad luck that his survival is one of the more amazing tales of human endurance and adaptation. You'll read about it in the last chapter.

I was able to visit Michael in Santa Fe in the winter of 2002, and, like people do, we talked about the good old days and how big a difference *The Book of Floating* had made to the floatation tank world, and how much we missed it. I thought of it first, "Why don't we republish?" There are so many more people floating now than there were in 1984 when the book first came out. Surely the tank centers around the world would offer this book to those coming to float and reading the book would help to expand the numbers of floaters.

Michael wanted to add a new chapter and when you read this new chapter

-—it's the last one,—you'll see the intensity of this addition. Read it many times! He put his email address at the end of this chapter so you can get in touch with him..

Michael wanted a new chapter, and I wanted a new cover. I didn't like the last cover and besides, I had the perfect picture for a great new cover. I inherited a Huichol yarn painting from my friend and mentor, Dr. John Lilly. It is the work of a Huichol shaman who floated in Dr. Lilly's tank and it shows a box with someone floating in it and representations of the symbols he saw while floating, made in the traditional patterns used in Huichol art.

I brought a photo of the art to the publisher to ask their approval for the cover. They loved the image, thought it would make a good cover and all that was needed was written permission of the artist and of course I would be the one to get it.

I was stopped. It seemed outrageously impossible! The Huichol live in uncharted territory in the mountains of Mexico and no one who is not Huichol can go there. I had the name of the shaman and no other clues. No one in the Lilly family knew anything about him nor did any close friends. Michael finished writing the new chapter and I worried about the cover art.

Right around that time it just so happened that I had arranged to meet Crash, owner of a new tank business on Venice Beach. He showed us his place, introduced us to his friend Margarita and we got down to "shop talk" which included republishing this book and the problem we were having with the cover.

You're probably guessing that some amazing coincidence is about to be revealed because first—you've already seen the cover—and next, we're dealing with the floatation tank, Dr. John Lilly's invention, and of course coincidence control is about to take over.

Margarita tells us that she is of Huichol ancestry and in fact her grandmother still lives in the Huichol community in Mexico and she would be happy to help. I got the feeling I always get when a miracle strikes. Very still, very quiet, out of time, deep breaths and a sense that all is well. What are the odds for a coincidence like that to happen?

A while later Margarita confessed to being a lawyer which allowed us great ease in preparing the contract to allow the art to be used for the cover. She began the search for Mr. Carrillo with her family's help. It was arranged that her family would go to Mexico with the papers to have them signed.

Margarita wrote about her parents' trip:

"He was about to take a bus to a very remote town and he would be inaccessible for at least 10 days. Alarmed by the news, my parents, aunts, uncles and grandma rushed to the bus station like a pack of crazy people. Whistling, shouting and waving, they finally caught up to Mr. Carrillo at the terminal just as he was boarding the bus. They got him off the bus, explained who they were, read him the letter, obtained his signature on all the copies and took his picture.

"My family had loads of fun the entire time!

IT WAS A GREAT MIRACLE ALL THE WAY AROUND!"

So I hope that this lucky book signals a change in luck for Michael Hutchison. Here's to the best of luck to Michael and to all the readers of this book.

—Lee Perry
President, Samadhi Tank Co., Inc.
www.samadhitank.com

INTRODUCTION
STEPPING INTO THE PRIVATE SEA

This is a book about floating atop a ten-inch-deep pool of water in a dark, enclosed chamber about the size of a small closet lying on its side. The book will present a lot of evidence that this practice is not only fun but very good for you.

Much of the information here is based on the current work of and interviews with experimental psychologists, neuroscientists, physicians, and others engaged in research into the effects of float tanks. In many cases this material is being made public for the first time. In the following pages you will learn:

≈ About indications that floating stimulates the brain to secrete endorphins: pain-killing, euphoria-creating substances known as the "body's own opiates."

≈ That there is evidence that tank use not only can initiate substantial weight loss but also has an unprecedented maintenance effect, with weight loss continuing at the same degree for many months after floating.

≈ Of evidence that floating results in a spontaneous reduction in or elimination of such habits as smoking, drinking, and drug use, and counteracts addiction withdrawal symptoms.

≈ That laboratory studies show that floating can rapidly and significantly decrease stress and anxiety, by sharply lowering the levels of biochemicals directly related to stress, anxiety, tension, the "fight or flight response," and heart disease and other stress-related illnesses.

≈ About indications that floating can suspend the dominance of the detail-oriented left hemisphere of the brain, allowing the right hemisphere (which deals with large-scale and novel information) to operate freely, giving the floater access to unusual powers of creativity, imagination, visualization, and problem solving.

≈ How athletes use floatation to improve their performance significantly, to speed their recovery from the stress of peak output, and virtually to eliminate fatigue and "post-race letdown."

≈ How floatation tanks are being used in schools and universities as tools for "superlearning," increasing the mind's powers of comprehension, retention, and original thinking.

≈ Of indications that two hours of floating are more restful and restorative than a full night of sound sleep, making floating, in the words of one prominent scientist, "a method of attaining the deepest rest that we have ever experienced."

Powerful claims. Yet these are only a few of the beneficial results attributed to floating. As word of floating's impressive effects begins to circulate, increasing numbers of researchers in laboratories, clinics, hospitals, universities, and float centers around the world are exploring a wide range of uses for floatation tanks—from overcoming snake phobias, stage fright, gastrointestinal disorders, and chronic anxiety, to breaking world athletic records. And as tank research has intensified in recent months, researchers seem on the threshold of even more dramatic breakthroughs.

So it was with a sense of urgency, excitement, and a widely shared belief that floating had reached a "critical mass" that more than one hundred scientists and researchers with a special interest in the use of float tanks—clinical and experimental psychologists, educators, neuroscientists, endocrinologists, biofeedback authorities, psychiatrists, therapists, commercial float-center operators, tank manufacturers—gathered in Denver for the First International Conference on REST and Self-Regulation, in the spring of 1983. (REST is an acronym for "Restricted Environmental Stimulation Technique," which refers to the use of float tanks and isolation chambers.)

While scientists had been working with sensory deprivation and floatation tanks for years, the Denver conference marked the first time authorities from such a wide range of backgrounds and scholarly disciplines had convened. They exchanged information and speculations, making new connections between areas of specialization, with a growing awareness that the range and power of the effects of floating were far greater than any single researcher had imagined. All agreed that the time had arrived when floatation tanks could no longer be considered mere curiosities confined to university psych labs, a hundred or two commercial float centers, and the spare bedrooms of a few thousand devotees. It was time to acknowledge the tanks' astonishing versatility, as essential equipment for clinics, hospitals, schools, health and fitness centers, gymnasiums, stress-management centers, offices, factories, prisons, addiction treatment centers, country clubs, hotels, resorts, spas, homes.

If you are a bit dubious about all these claims of remarkable and life-enhancing effects, that's understandable. I started out a skeptic myself. The whole thing seemed so *California*, so of a piece with hot tubs, Baba Free Rubadub, and psychobabble. My home is Manhattan, and New Yorkers take great pleasure in scoffing at all things Californian—i.e., softheaded, mellow, self-indulgent, healthy. So when I heard about a tank center in New York, I spoke to the editor of a weekly magazine reputed for its contentious and cantankerous style of journalism, proposing that I do an article on "the whole phenomenon." She allowed that the concept sounded amusing, but just so I knew I wasn't to take this thing seriously, she said, "Remember, we don't want a puff piece—this thing should have an edge to it."

"Right," said I, "an edge to it."

I was fully ready to see float tanks as another example of America's inability to distinguish the sublime from the ridiculous, its tendency to approach spiritual goals through inappropriate technological means: drag-racing to paradise. I had read of one tank manufacturer's ambition for his company to be "the Big Mac of mind expansion." I had no doubt there was an edge to be found.

And yet something about the idea had beckoned me in the first place, had made me actively seek the article assignment. As I thought back, I realized I'd been drawn to the idea ever since I'd first heard about Dr. John Lilly's float tank experiments in the sixties. In my mind for years had been a picture of an isolation tank: a huge, black, whale-like machine humming in some dank underground laboratory, wires running to a bank of chattering machines with blinking lights, wild-eyed scientists running around clutching clipboards and muttering about EELs, as some wombed-out explorer of inner-space floated silently within the box, blissful and wrinkled like a prune. It all seemed quite interesting, intriguing even, but exotic, expensive, far removed from the vicissitudes of daily urban life.

Then along came the movie *Altered States*—a young scientist climbs into the mysterious tank and emerges shortly as a screeching hairy ape with an appetite for live gazelle. Bloodlust, running naked through the streets. What fun. In what seemed like only a few months, I'd begun to hear about these tanks in trend-testing places like Aspen, Tucson, Fort Lauderdale, San Francisco, L.A.—commercial floatation tank centers where anyone could walk in off the street and rent an hour as an inner-space cowboy, something like trampoline centers, GoKart tracks or theme adventure parks. A magazine for entrepreneurs named a float tank manufacturer as "one of the one hundred best investments in the world." New centers were opening all over.

But something about this puzzled me: curious, these millions paying $20 a pop to be absolutely alone for an hour or two—precious loneliness!—in a culture where most are so terrified of being alone they'll drop $20 just to sit around a bar with people they can't stand. How retrograde, these masses paying enthusiastically to enter a state of "sensory deprivation" in a culture where status is earned by frantically exposing one's senses to as many stimulations as possible (and as conspicuously as possible). The phenomenon fascinated me. Where's the thrill, I wondered, in lying all alone in a box? Then I heard that there was a float center just a few blocks from me, and it occurred to me that this was something I would like to try myself.

Actually, I was quite eager to float, but as a somewhat starving writer drenched in the work ethic I could never allow myself to pay $20 an hour to float merely for my own enlightenment and pleasure. Not only was it too expensive, it smacked of self-indulgence, narcissism—that is, California. But with an expense account from the magazine to pay for a whole series of floats—purely as "research" of course—I could indulge myself with a clear conscience: After all, I was a journalist, boldly seeking out new experiences and information, floating not because I wanted to but because it was an *assignment.* And all I had to do was make sure there was an edge to it.

And so I found myself standing wet, naked, and alone one afternoon, preparing to climb into what looked like a giant wooden coffin with one beveled end. The tank, operated by Tranquility Tanks in a loft eight floors above lower Fifth Avenue in Manhattan, was in a pleasant private room; soft lights played through prisms casting rainbows along the walls, a bouquet of lilacs adorned the tank, and the room had its own shower, toiletries—everything one might conceivably need for hours of luxurious floating. And yet, despite the pleasant surroundings, the fact remained: The damn thing was like a coffin, and dark inside, and I felt a little edgy about crawling into it.

I had determined to go through with the float before talking to anyone experienced, so that my reactions would be free of expectations and of someone else's ideas, but I *had* heard somewhere that tanks were absolutely safe for everyone but "borderline" cases. Was I, unbeknownst to myself, on some psychic border, so that a few jolts of sensory deprivation would send me climbing over the wire, to emerge from the tank drooling and goggle-eyed, babbling of aliens who had communicated to me a special message that would save the world? With an overpowering hunger for live gazelle? Later, in talking with floaters, I discovered that almost everyone feels a few whim-whams the first time in the tank: *Will I be able to breathe? Will I drown? Will I feel claustrophobic?* In fact, it's probably part of our genetic heritage, this canny reluctance to insert oneself into a tiny, pitch-black, soundproof enclosure filled with water—and if it isn't, it should be.

But once inside the tank, the edginess translated into excitement. I was ready for a taste of the millennium. I stretched out on my back; the water was only ten inches deep, but saturated with eight hundred pounds of Epsom salts; it had such buoyancy, I bobbed on top of it like a rubber duckie in a giant bathtub. I reached up, pulled the hatch shut, and was instantly in a different place: utter blackness. *I've never seen anything this black in my entire life,* said a voice in my head.

The water, warmed to a constant 93.5 degrees Fahrenheit, felt neither warm nor cool, and very quickly seemed to disappear altogether, leaving me with the feeling of floating weightlessly on my back in black space. The absence of external stimuli turned my awareness inward, and I realized there is no such thing as sensory deprivation: I was creating my own sensory stimulation. My stomach gurgled like a cement mixer, my heart boomed, my lungs wheezed like bellows, and my eyeballs danced with colors, pinwheels of light. Slowly my body seemed to spin, as if I were riding a huge whirlpool. My body seemed to rise from horizontal to vertical and continued to rotate until I seemed to be floating belly-down and weightless in black starless space, with no vertigo or discomfort. *Okay,* said the voice in my head, *so it's a body trip.*

Not so, or not entirely so. As each part of my body became deeply relaxed, that part seemed to disappear from awareness. The heart and lung sounds went away and my body evaporated, until there was nothing left but me. At some point in the next hour there came a series of what I can only call "events," a seamless intermingling of ideas, images, sounds, sensations, emotions. My memory tossed up odd chunks—childhood scenes, vivid but fragmentary—which merged with familiar faces speaking to me, bright fantasies, shorthand thought notation that passed for ideas. They occurred helter-skelter, and were a lot of fun. I decided to try to control the stream of events and found I could do so—like directing my own movie. However, the effort of will it took to control things seemed to distract me from the mindless pleasures of merely circulating. I decided just to let go....

After what seemed like only a few minutes, peaceful electronic music gurgled into my ears from underwater speakers-the signal that my hour was up. As I sank back into a heavy body from somewhere far away, the voice in my head spoke quite distinctly: *They're going to have to come in and get me.*

I chuckled and stretched deliciously in the silky water, and the voice spoke again: *Next time I'll stay longer.* This made me laugh. I felt an immensely pleasant lassitude, similar to but better than that period after the alarm clock goes off and you continue to doze, half awake in bed. And yet I was somehow disappointed. Was this all it was? Nice, relaxing, some good sensations, but $20 worth? I was disappointed because I assumed the ride was over. I was mistaken. As I opened the hatch and climbed out I began to discover that the float is just the beginning; it's what happens afterward that can be the most stunning part of the process.

As I stand upright, my muscles are heavy but feel good—maybe something like an astronaut returning to gravity after a short time in space. Why do I keep chuckling deep in my throat, I wonder? I look at myself in the mirror—ten years younger and a lot happier than when I went in—and burst out laughing. O sun-kissed youthling! In the shower my skin is sleek, and it gives me pleasure to touch it. I find I am singing loudly, and shake my head from side to side, laughing.

On Fifth Avenue in the late afternoon light, I am made aware of how acute all my senses have become. My vision is sharp, all images clear, the colors intense. I smell everything, eagerly; as women pass by I scent each one from yards away, fragrance wafting from them and hanging in the air long after they've passed. An endless parade of beauty! My ears are so keen I'm overwhelmed, keeping track of eight or ten conversations going on around me, some as much as half a block away. The conversations strike me as sparklingly witty or absurdly comical, and I can't keep a silly grin off my face. I run into a friend, and when we kiss I get a sudden intense whiff of tobacco; my lips sting from the nicotine on hers. Crossing Fourteenth Street I'm stunned by a blast of cheap cigar smoke, hot dogs, late spring air, masses of people, and I am whirled back to the first time my dad took me out to the ball park. And all the while, I'm full of a calm, clear energy. *So,* says the voice in my head, *now we know what this floating-in-the-tank thing is all about.*

The feeling of being relaxed, recharged, and extremely sensitive went on for two days before tapering off. I began to talk with others who had floated, and found they'd all experienced a similar intensification of sensations after coming out of the tank. Many mentioned increased sexual pleasure. They said they looked younger, thought better, worked better. Obviously, I thought, something that makes you feel so good has to be illegal, immoral, or fattening.

I wondered, are these effects *real,* or do I only *feel* that they're real? Is there a difference? What I needed was empirical verification, scientific knowledge, not the ecstatic hymns of fellow floaters. I began talking with scientists who had impeccable reputations and who had done years of research into sensory deprivation, and found that floating did indeed create a whole range of "beneficial disturbances" in perceptions, including the enhancement of learning, recall, I.Q. scores, visual concentration, visual storage, and various perceptual-motor tasks.

My interviews with research scientists led me into talks with tank manufacturers, operators of float centers, tank designers, consultants on health and fitness, and professional athletes who used the tank for improving their "inner game"; over and over I found that where I'd expected to hear ethereal effusions about cosmic vibrations, I found instead everyone speaking in down-to-earth language about specific uses for tanks, ways of using tanks as a "tool" (a favorite word with all tank people). Everyone I spoke to believed that the time was fast approaching when tanks would come into everyday use, as educational, therapeutic, and recreational tools. One man even confided to me that he thought the tank would have a transforming effect on all aspects of society. "Like television," he said, "but bigger."

Bigger than television! The idea was staggering and somehow unsettling. Visions of utopia always have ominous overtones. For decades most Americans went to the neighborhood theater frequently; it was a communal experience, sitting in a darkened room with hundreds of neighbors and strangers, sharing the same fantasy. If they didn't like what was playing, they had to wait a few days until the double feature changed. Then television came along—The Box—and the audience was reduced to individual families, sitting in darkened living rooms, who, if they didn't like what was playing, could change channels. Soon there were multiple-television families, and while the audience was reduced to one, the number of channels was increased (thanks to the cable hookup) to twenty, eighty, a hundred.

And now the tank, and people are finding they can leave behind not just neighbors and families and living rooms, but their own bodies. They don't *watch* the box, they *climb inside* it. And the movies they make in the dark are all their own, no commercials, and the channels are infinite, so if they don't like what's playing, they can, well, *change....*

But though I was fascinated by floaters, and had begun floating regularly myself, I assumed that these visions of mass popularity for tanks were just the product of their overheated enthusiasm. I went ahead and wrote my article—discovering for the first but not the last time that the tank is a valuable tool for a free-lance writer: The night before my deadline for the floating article I still had no idea of what I would write, so I took a long float during which the article took shape in an instant, and I rushed home to type it up word for word with my hair still wet.

So it was with some surprise that I observed the extraordinary response to the article. The float centers I mentioned in the article were instantly overwhelmed with calls and letters from all over the United States asking for appointments to float, and for the addresses of local tanks. Inquiries came from all over the world, and vacationers or business travelers from Europe would stop in to float because of the article. The Manhattan center was quickly booked solid for four months in advance. The enthusiastic response went on and on, and soon where there had been only the two tanks of Tranquility Tanks in Manhattan, there were more than thirty tanks available commercially in numerous settings, ranging from a Soho beauty salon to the physical-fitness-oriented Biofitness Institute.

I began talking with floaters from all over the country. They introduced me to friends who floated, who introduced me to other friends.... Most of them at one point or another told me that floating had changed their lives. They were not exaggerating. They told me remarkable tales of how they had overcome depression, alcoholism, recurrent panic attacks, lifelong shyness, or chronic fatigue, and had become more creative, happier, healthier, loving, energetic.

To such tales the still-strong skeptic crouched within me said, *well, maybe there really IS something to this floating stuff!* I began conducting interviews and doing research in earnest, trying to find out as much as I could about floating. I discovered that no one had ever approached the subject in a comprehensive and systematic way. I decided to do it myself.

The result is this book, which is not only *about* floating, but was conceived while floating and largely written in my mind while floating. In general, it has the shape of a float, starting out from the factual, the historical, plunging into the sensual immediacy of the experience, emerging into the real world once again but somehow made different, and with the determination to find out more about the whole process.

In Part I, we will look at the long history of sensory deprivation as a tool for altering the human mind and body, culminating in the invention of the modern float tank.

In Part II, we will try to find out just what makes the floating experience unique and powerful, isolating the mechanisms by which the tank works, dividing them into a number of separate "explanations" or useful paradigms.

In Part III, we will see how the extraordinary effects of the tank can be harnessed, directed, and applied to a wide range of practical situations. We will emerge to an Appendix of practical information helpful to those who want to learn more about floating and perhaps to buy or build their own tank. (The Bibliography that follows the Appendix is numbered; corresponding superscript numbers entered in the text refer the interested reader to the sources of quotations and research projects described.)

Since the book is structured like a float, it's my hope that you'll immerse yourself in it, floating gently, ruminatively, with bemused detachment and unhurried pleasure through its pages, pausing now and then to consider, making connections, flowing on, and finally emerging with a changed sense of your own powers; a changed awareness of what is possible, probable, desirable; a changed perception of the world you inhabit, the life you live.

But however pleasant the float provided by this book may be, it cannot substitute for the true float, the silent, weightless float in the utter dark of the tank. That book of floating is the one you write yourself.

PART I

A SHORT HISTORY
OF THE FLOAT

... it is easier to sail many thousands of miles through cold and storm and cannibals, in a government ship, with five hundred men and boys to assist one, than it is to explore the private sea, the Atlantic and Pacific Ocean of one's being alone.

—H. D. THOREAU, **Walden**

They were anchorites, i.e., withdrawers, because being by no means satisfied with that victory whereby they had trodden underfoot the hidden snares of the devil (while still living among men), they were eager to fight with the devil in open conflict and straightforward battle, and so feared not to penetrate the vast recesses of the desert.

—JOHN CASSIAN, **Colloquia**

Was that what travel meant? An exploration of the deserts of memory, rather than those around me?

—CLAUDE LÉVI-STRAUSS, **Tristes Tropiques**

ONE

LESS IS MORE—THE SENSORY RESTRICTION TRADITION

The Discovery of the Blind Pew Effect

I was about four when I had my first experience of the nature of sensory deprivation. My father was reading me Robert Louis Stevenson's *Treasure Island*. We'd reached the exciting chapter in which Jim Hawkins and the sea captain are seated in the Admiral Benbow Inn; suddenly Pew, a blind beggar, comes in, finding his way hesitantly, tapping a cane, until he reaches the captain, whereupon he gives him a message bearing the dreaded Black Spot and races out of the inn. "But wait", I said: "How can this blind man, who could barely find his way into the inn without tripping over chairs and tables, now race out of the tavern so easily?" My father explained that blind people, because they had to rely on senses other than sight, were able to develop those other senses to a very high degree. Blind Pew, he assured me, could certainly find his way out of any place he entered, because as he found his way in he was unconsciously visualizing the floor plan in his head. It is, he said, like a sixth sense.

I immediately decided I would keep my eyes shut and pretend I was blind until I could make use of that sixth sense. In the coming days I spent a lot of time stumbling into chairs, tripping over curbs, and sitting in the total darkness of an empty refrigerator box I'd discovered in the garbage, but no matter how hard I tried I couldn't seem to generate that elusive inner sense. Then, while sitting in the coal bin in the basement, I realized that I was anticipating the tuna casserole mother was making for dinner. Hold on—I hadn't even known what she was cooking! Then I understood that real knowledge had come to me unconsciously through my nose and ears. Excitedly I paid attention, heard my mother talking to herself upstairs, and every pot clanking, every floorboard squeaking, every odor took on meaning. I could visualize her every movement. I was the blind Pew of my coal cellar! I could hear the sounds, and from the sounds create an inner vision: of my friends playing stickball amid the traffic outside and flipping baseball cards on the front stoop, my sisters chattering as they put on their roller skates, the baseball game on the radio from across the street. The world was going on outside me, and without seeing it I could experience it inside me more clearly than I usually did with my eyes open ... and suddenly I opened my eyes.

There I was in the dim cellar sitting on a pile of hard coal. Somehow the sounds seemed to have been turned down; all the richness and timeless complexity of the noise of a whole neighborhood went away. But I was thrilled. I had an image of my mind as something like a balloon—if you squeezed it in one place it swelled up someplace else. I had made a discovery that must be one of the first every child makes, and one of the earliest realizations of our ancient ancestors: *When one or more senses are restricted, the sensitivity of the other senses is expanded.*

Such experiences are probably universal. Dr. Andrew Weil believes they flow from an innate human drive. As he wrote in *The Natural Mind*: "Human beings are born with a drive to experience modes of awareness other than the normal waking one; from very young ages, children experiment with techniques to change consciousness. Such experiences are normal."

But though this universal drive to alter consciousness is a source of great pleasure to children, it is not mere child's play. Weil sees it as "evolutionary," representing an "innate capacity of the nervous system," and concludes: "It is valuable to learn to enter other states deliberately and consciously because such experiences are doorways to fuller use of the nervous system, to the realization of untapped human potential, and to better function in the ordinary mode of consciousness."

This need to alter consciousness, then, is not some frivolous desire to escape, but rather one of the most fundamental of human characteristics— perhaps, in fact, the characteristic that has led to our development of culture and civilization. The point is at once so obvious, so important, and so easily forgotten: To be human is to explore and make use of altered states of consciousness.

Probably the most satisfactory and popular way of altering consciousness—a method that humans have developed over literally millions of years of testing and exploring—is to restrict the operation of one or more of their senses, that is, to put themselves into a state of sensory deprivation. One of the main assumptions of this book is that the floatation tank makes use of this sensory deprivation effect to bring about a gentle, pleasant, controllable, and temporary shift in consciousness in anyone who floats. Among the ideas proposed here is that this shift in consciousness is healthy, that it is educational, and that it can be manipulated, explored, and used in such a way as to cause changes in attitude, physiology, and behavior that persist even after one emerges from the tank.

Floating in Artist's Garret, Polar Icecap, and Monk's Cell

The float tank is a valuable specific tool for cutting down the amount of external stimuli that reach our senses, probably the best sensory deprivation device ever created. But humans have been using tools and techniques of various sorts for exactly this purpose for thousands, probably millions of years. The following are just a few of the most common:

Preparation for the Hunt. In primitive societies, like those our own civilization has evolved from, men prepare themselves before going out on a hunt by withdrawing from normal activities and "purifying" themselves through fasting, silence, steam baths, and/or isolation, either within a small shelter or alone in some spot away from village life. They believe that this sensory restriction improves their hunting abilities; and recent tests, demonstrating that short periods of sensory deprivation increase acuity of smell, taste, sight, and hearing, show that the ancient hunters knew what they were doing.

Rites of Passage. In every premodern society an important ceremony marks the passage from childhood to acceptance into adult society. These rites of passage gain much of their power from the inclusion of more or less arduous sensory deprivation as part of the preparation. Some young people are confined for days or weeks to darkened huts, or undertake fasts. In many cultures the boys are expected to go out alone into the wilderness for long periods until they have experienced their spiritual coming of age, by confronting demons, ghosts, ancestral spirits, or dreams—the dream quest. Whatever the sensory deprivation technique used, it works in part by making the young people more open to new experience, new wisdom, new responsibility, by making them more sensitive and aware, so that the experiences they undergo will be intensified, momentous, unforgettable.

Spiritual Withdrawal. In every culture some sort of sensory deprivation experience has been considered essential in the training of spiritual leaders. Shamans, witch doctors, monks, priests, gurus, fakirs, yogis, priestesses, mediums, mystics, and other spiritual seekers endure frequent and often rigorous periods of total silence, fasting, retreat into small cells or caves or dark rooms, withdrawal to mountaintops or deserts or islands where isolation can be combined with restricted or monotonous sensory input. Like the desert anchorites or "withdrawers" mentioned by John Cassian in the quotation that opened this section, hermits, monks, and seekers of enlightenment have always found sensory restriction—either the actual isolation of desert, monastery, or cave; or the mental equivalent of such isolation, attained through concentrative/restrictive meditation and prayer techniques—an important part of all mystical, transcendental, or revelatory states.

Spiritual Practices.   Similar restrictions of attention have been painstakingly recorded by medieval alchemists, in their endless repetitions of grinding and distillation of various chemical compounds.   The record of their attempts to transform ordinary base materials by means of the philosophers' stone into alchemical gold is also, we now know, a symbolic description of their attempts to transform ordinary consciousness through various sensory deprivation techniques into the higher levels of awareness, symbolized by gold. You could make a sizable list of craftsmen and workers of all sorts who have used intense concentration on seemingly mundane tasks to restrict their senses for spiritual or pleasurable purposes—including craftsmen who carve long scriptural passages on tiny pieces of ivory, weavers, calligraphers, jewelers, silversmiths, tailors, and so on.

Creative Isolation.   Numerous profound aesthetic experiences, and moments of creative illumination, insight, or revelation have occurred in circumstances in which sensory input has been reduced in some way. We all know stories of artists or scientists whose sudden creative intuitions or revelations have come to them in the confines of the "artist's garret" or while staring into the fireplace or walking on the beach with attention turned inward. In fact, one of the essential elements of all creative thought is concentration gained through some sort of restriction of sensory stimulation.

Involuntary Isolation.   There are many fascinating accounts by people who have experienced involuntary sensory isolation, often for long periods—polar explorers lost for months in a white void, solitary sailors, shipwreck or aircrash survivors, prisoners confined to isolation cells, desert explorers. And virtually all of them speak of some enlightening transformation brought about by sensory deprivation.

Isolation on the Couch.   One of the greatest values of traditional psychotherapy derives from its sensory deprivation effect: As the patient reclines in a relaxed position (with the analyst, usually silent, sitting behind) there is little visual or auditory stimulus to distract the patient from a free-associative, almost trancelike state.

Getting Away from It All. Modern urban dwellers place great value on having a place at the shore or a cabin in the mountains. Conspicuous consumption, someone might sniff, but these hideaways are looked on as near necessities: The sensory overload of city life requires recovery periods, and clinical studies of stress have now shown conclusively that temporary infusions of the peace, quiet, and solitude of mountain, forest, ocean, or country are essential for maintaining health and sanity.

This list of various forms of sensory isolation that mankind has found useful, essential, or pleasurable could be extended to include sleep, naps, hypnosis, games, reverie, daydreaming, deep involvement in reading or listening to music, repetitive exercise such as jogging, and so on. But it should be clear by now that the use of sensory isolation has a long and respectable history, and should not be viewed as mere escapism. Sensory restriction is an effective way of turning *toward* reality, of *increasing* our sensitivity to and awareness of the world as it is.

Altered states of consciousness have been found to share a number of general characteristics, among them alterations in thinking, changes in the sense of time, changes in body image, a sense of the ineffable, feelings of rejuvenation, hypersuggestibility, change in emotional expression, and temporary release from ego control. These are also cardinal characteristics of the float experience, as we shall see later. But for now let us just divide the tank experience into two parts: what happens to you while you're in the tank, and what happens afterward.

In the Tank

Simply stated, when we shut out or restrict environmental stimuli, we become more aware of those things that are still available to us. In this case, after we have shut out light, sound, tactile sensations, gravity, other people, and movement, what is left is our Self: the physical reality of our skeletal muscles, our internal systems, our brains; and the non-physical reality of our thoughts, emotions, intuitions, mental images. Our awareness of these realities is of a subtlety and intensity simply not possible when our senses are directed outward, responding to external events.

This intensified awareness is not some contentless or other-worldly state, of little use in the "real world." Scientists from many disciplines have accumulated overwhelming evidence that by becoming more acutely cognizant of their inner processes, humans can actually exercise conscious control over them. For example, experiments show that simply by focusing awareness inward in a certain way, a person can actually strengthen his or her immune system, lower blood pressure, slow the heartbeat, release or inhibit the release of hormones, alleviate pain, cause parts of the body to grow or shrink, and alter the activity of the heart, muscles, brain, and mind.

The discovery that humans can control their own bodies through alertness to subtle internal signals was made largely by researchers using biofeedback techniques, and is certainly one of the most astounding scientific developments of the last fifteen years. However, it is really nothing very new. Using sensory deprivation techniques, yogis, monks, and fakirs have been performing these "miracles" of self-regulation for thousands of years, in blithe ignorance of our Western scientists who said such things could not be done. We need think only of Hindu fire walkers; of Tibetan monks who, through meditative techniques, raise their body temperature so that they can sit, in subzero snow, and dry scores of wet, icy blankets wrapped around them; of Yogis who are buried alive for days in airtight boxes; of healers and mystics who can puncture themselves with knitting needles yet experience no pain and whose bodies heal almost instantly.

Few of us have much desire to puncture ourselves with knitting needles, and I have rarely felt an urgent need to dry forty ice-water-soaked sheets upon my naked body while sitting in a snowbank, but the "secret" of these and other forms of seemingly miraculous self-regulation is increased awareness of internal processes. That it can be quite a useful secret is attested to by all those sufferers who have learned to alleviate crippling migraine headaches by consciously increasing the blood flow to their hands, and by "terminal" cancer patients who, using techniques based on sensory deprivation, have learned to become aware of their internal states and to visualize their bodies eradicating the disease, resulting in complete recovery.

At the heart of what happens in the tank, then, is a paradox: By restricting sensory input, we increase sensory awareness; by becoming blind, we learn to see in a new and more powerful way; by giving up, letting go, we gain greater control and power over ourselves and, ultimately, over the external world.

Out of the Tank

If merely being in the tank can increase your awareness of even the most minute internal processes, the increase in awareness that occurs after you get out of the tank is no less profound. People who emerge from the tank are often delighted to find that the world seems to have changed while they were away. They speak of seeing things anew, and describe the world as fresh, glowing, illuminated, bright, intensified, more vivid, luminous, and so on. The Blind Pew Effect comes into play full force: When you cut down on the input to your senses by going into the tank, your senses seem to respond by expanding, becoming more sensitive. William Blake described the process as "cleansing the doors of perception." Zen masters talk about seeing the world with a "beginner's mind." Jesus spoke of the need to see with the fresh perceptions of a child. Psychologists have called it "deautomatization."

Whatever the terminology, after floating we seem to perceive the world with startling directness, richness, and clarity. And whatever the spiritual value of this kind of perception, we know immediately that it is worth having simply because it feels so good. Ultimately, whatever other virtues we may find in the float tanks this is the one we will come back to again and again: It is a rapid, easily mastered, reliable, safe tool to make you feel very good.

TWO

THE DEVELOPMENT OF
THE FLOATATION TANK

While various forms of sensory deprivation have been used for thousands of years by children, artists, mystics, yogis, monks, mothers, and others, for purposes of peace, pleasure, propagation, meditation, relief from stress, relaxation, enlightenment, and just plain fun, it was—appropriately enough for our scientific, brain-obsessed age—a scientist of the brain who developed the floatation tank. When he first set about creating a simple floatation tank, Dr. John C. Lilly, an M.D. with training as a psychoanalyst and a specialty in experimental neurophysiology, was not thinking about meditative states of consciousness, peace, or pleasure, but was trying to create what he calls "a research instrument" with which he could study some puzzling areas of neuropsychology.

For more than twenty years Lilly had been pursuing his studies of the brain, particularly its electrical activity. Fascinated by the seemingly unknowable connection between the physical brain and what is commonly known as mind, Lilly was determined to record objectively the electrical activity of the brain and the simultaneous, corresponding (and somehow related) activity and changes of thoughts, feelings, ideas. For over two decades, Lilly approached the mind-brain problem in a number of ways. He implanted electrodes in the brains of monkeys and began to map various areas in which electrical stimulation would prompt the monkey to various reactions. "I was seeking methods of objective fast recordings of the activities of the brain," says Lilly, "and, simultaneously, objective fast recordings of the activities of the mind in that brain."

After years of exploring the electrical activity of the brain, however, Lilly reluctantly concluded that there was no way of picking up and recording its activities without damaging and changing the brain, and thereby altering the mind that was contained in (or contained) the brain. While searching for a way to study the processes of brain/mind without changing or damaging it, Lilly also became intrigued by the related question of the origins of conscious

activity within the brain. There were at that time (the early 1950s) two
schools of thought on this question. In Lilly's words:

> The first school hypothesized that the brain needed stimulation
> from external reality to keep its conscious states going. This school
> maintained that sleep resulted as soon as the brain was freed of exter-
> nal stimulation.... The second school maintained that the activities of
> the brain were inherently autorhythmic; in other words, within the
> brain substance itself were cells that tended to continue their oscilla-
> tions without the necessity of any external stimuli. According to this
> interpretation, the origins of consciousness were in the natural rhythms
> of the brain's cell circuitry itself.[140]

In 1954, while working at the National Institutes of Mental Health
(NIMH), Lilly perceived that the way to approach *both* the problem of studying
the brain/mind and the question of the origins of consciousness was to isolate
the mind from external stimulation. Why isolation? As Lilly writes in his book
The Deep Self:

> My reasoning was founded on a basic tenet of certain experimental
> sciences (physics, biology, et cetera): in order to adequately study a sys-
> tem, all known influences to and from that system must either be atten-
> uated below threshold for excitation, reliably accounted for, or elimi-
> nated to avoid *unplanned disturbances* of that system. Disturbances from
> unknown sources may then be found and dealt with more adequately.[139]

Serendipitously, Lilly found that an ideal facility was available at the
National Institutes of Health—a soundproof chamber containing a tank con-
structed during World War II for experiments by the navy on the metabolism
of underwater swimmers. Lilly and his associate Jay Shurley, M.D., a
researcher in neuropsychiatry with particular interest in sensory deprivation,
set to work trying to devise a system that would restrict environmental stimulation as much as was practical and feasible.

Lilly's first tank was one in which the floater was suspended upright,
entirely underwater, head completely covered by a vividly ugly molded-rubber
underwater breathing apparatus and mask, and dangling like the Creature
from the Black Lagoon on the end of an air hose. Lilly found that the tank
effectively eliminated virtually all major external stimuli. Among these, the
most important were:

≈ *Other people.* No danger of meeting someone else floating in your tank, so no need to worry about social roles, what you look like, or who might interrupt you.

≈ *Light.* By covering the entire head with an opaque helmet, Lilly sealed out all external light—total blackout, a condition rarely if ever experienced in normal life.

≈ *Sound.* Noise does not pass well from air into water, so the floater was in a state of almost total silence.

≈ *Gravity.* A large proportion of our energy (some physiologists estimate as much as 85 percent) and much of our brain is devoted to dealing with and counteracting gravity. Eliminating the body's specific gravity by suspending it in water also eliminated an inexorable, powerful, and constant external stimulation, liberating large regions of the mind and great quantities of energy for novel purposes.

≈ *Temperature.* Temperature has a great effect on us: If it is too cold, the body responds with tension and shivering; heat causes us to sweat. The body constantly reacts to temperature, and we deal with it in part by wearing clothes that enhance comfort in the prevailing climate. With experimentation, Lilly and Shurley found that heating the water in the tank to a steady 93.5 degrees Fahrenheit caused it to be experienced as neither warm nor cold but neutral, and after a few minutes the consciousness of relative temperature disappeared completely.

After designing the tank, the next step was to try it out, and Lilly and Shurley had no hesitation in choosing their experimental subjects: themselves. At that time, 1954, this was something of a step into the unknown. The Korean War had recently ended, and both the American public and the scientific community were being flooded with shocking stories of American prisoners of war who had been subjected to "brainwashing" techniques, among them sensory deprivation. These stories were later shown to be myths, but at the time, many looked on sensory isolation as a particularly horrifying type of Chinese water torture. At the same time, people were quite interested in finding out just how sensory deprivation worked. Because of the new threat of the Cold War, we now had many soldiers staring into radar screens for hours at a time, scanning for the blip that meant missiles were coming at us over the pole. But these radar watchers were experiencing strange symptoms: disorientation, trances, hallucinations. It wouldn't do to have one of these lads hallucinate a fusillade of Russky nukes across the Distant Early

Warning line, since such a delusion could turn into a self-fulfilling prophecy. Similarly, as our military forces experimented with high-altitude jet flights, they were finding that at great heights, where there was nothing really to see, the test pilots were experiencing what they called "break-off" phenomena, suddenly losing all interest in earthly things like controlling the airplane or reporting back to base, but sliding into strange, euphoric states of mind, god-like amusement at the thought of the poor little mortals struggling away so far below. If this happened at just 50,000 feet, what might happen to the first astronaut? Clearly, we needed to do some study of this whole sensory deprivation problem.

The most influential study of isolation that had as yet been carried out was the work of Dr. Donald Hebb's Department of Psychology at McGill University. The 1953 study had focused on monotonous stimulation rather than reduced stimulation, by placing the subjects immobile on a bed inside an air-conditioned isolation chamber, arms and gloved hands swathed in cardboard sleeve restraints, eyes covered, the chambers filled with diffuse light and white noise. The subjects had been recruited (and were paid) for an experiment in "sensory deprivation," and had every reason to expect the negative experience promised by the word *deprivation*. They found it hard to think with organization or to maintain concentration for sustained periods. They became highly suggestible (thus reinforcing the experimenters' expectations about brainwashing possibilities). They grew nervous and anxious, and developed delusions and bizarre hallucinations. There were some seizures. In general, the McGill experiments fulfilled the negative expectations of the researchers.

So in the mid-fifties it was thought that sensory deprivation was a road to madness. Given such assumptions in the scientific community, Lilly must have felt some trepidation when he first immersed himself in the float tank, entering a state of deprivation that could perhaps drive him crazy, at best frighten and disorient him. We can imagine his surprise as he quickly found that the absence of external stimuli, rather than depriving him, instead projected him into what he calls "richly elaborate states of inner experience."

As for the classical puzzle about the origins of conscious activity in the brain—i.e., is the brain self-maintaining or in need of external stimulation?—Lilly writes (speaking of himself in the third person):

"Within the first few hours of exposure with satisfactory apparatus, he found out which school of thought was correct: the theory that the brain contained self-sustaining oscillators and did not need external forms of stimulation to stay conscious had been proven." [140] In fact, Lilly and Shurley concluded in an early article: "When given freedom from external exchanges and transactions, the isolated-constrained ego (or self or personality) has sources of *new information* from within." [142]

With that first float Lilly made an additional, surprising discovery: Rather than being stressful, the isolation experience was profoundly unstressful. As he writes of himself:

> The scientist made his second discovery: this environment furnished the most profound relaxation and rest that he had ever experienced in this life. It was far superior to a bed for purposes of recuperation from the stresses of the day's work.... He found that there were many, many states of consciousness, of being, between the usual wide-awake consciousness of participating in an external reality and the unconscious state of deep sleep. He found that he could have voluntary control of these states: that he could have, if he wished, waking dreams, hallucinations; total events could take place in the inner realities that were so brilliant and so "real" they could possibly be mistaken for events in the outside world. In this unique environment, freed of the usual sources of stimulation, he discovered that his mind and his central nervous system functioned in ways to which he had not yet accustomed himself. [140]

The scientific community, however, was not prepared for such a positive, almost evangelical attitude toward what they insisted on seeing as "psychopathological phenomena." Unable to gain acceptance for his ideas among academic scientists, Lilly continued his experiments with floatation, simplifying and improving the general design of the tank. He found that he could float in a more relaxing supine position, rather than suspended feet downward in fresh water, if the more-buoyant salt water was used. Finally he discovered that the best floatation was provided by a saturated solution of Epsom salts, which allowed even the thinnest of scientists to float with his entire body on or near the surface of the water. Other refinements, such as in-tank water heaters with thermostats sensitive enough to keep the water at perfect temperature, an air pump to keep the air in the tank fresh, and a water filter for the reuse of the Epsom salts solution, were added over the years.

By the early 1970s, Lilly had perfected the float tank in much the design popularly used today. Installing a number of these tanks in his Malibu home, Lilly—who had by then attained some notoriety through his attempts to communicate with dolphins and his investigations of inner space, recorded in such popular books as *The Mind of the Dolphin* and *The Center of the Cyclone*—began inviting influential members of the newly born "human potential" movement to try a float in his tanks. Influential gurus, culture leaders, artists, and authorities on "the mind game" stripped down and climbed into the vessels for an experience of "psychological free-fall" in "a black hole in psychophysical space." Figures such as Gregory Bateson, Werner Erhard, and many others came to float and found the tank an extraordinary toy and tool for exploring states of consciousness. They then wrote and/or spoke to others about the tanks, broadcasting the information in a widening ripple effect.

Many of these people had a lot of experience with meditation. They knew that to reach deep levels of meditation took much practice, repeated and sometimes frustrating efforts to shut out sounds, light, and other environmental stimuli. But the tank, they discovered, virtually eliminated these distractions, enabling them to go almost immediately to deep levels of meditation. In Lilly's words, the tank's "'reduced' environment allows one to start the meditation at the point only achievable *outside* the tank after some inhibitory work and some time spent doing that work. In the tank one need not do that work. Undistracted, one starts concentrating immediately upon one's inner perceptions and dives deep into one's mind." [139]

Many of Lilly's guests emerged feeling that they would like to repeat the experience every day and eager to obtain tanks of their own. At that time a young computer engineer, Glenn Perry, came to one of Lilly's float sessions. As Perry recently remembered it, he had always suffered from acute shyness: "I could never talk with more than one person at a time." After his first float Lilly asked him to address the group, and he did so with no discomfort. "For me," says the ebullient Perry, "that was *in-credible!* I immediately had to have my own tank." Using his engineering skills, Perry designed and built a tank that was inexpensive and relatively easy to build and maintain. Lilly made use of Perry's tank design. The word began to spread, and more and more of Perry's tanks were installed in the homes of people who had discovered floating through an experience at Lilly's place. Perry met and married Lee Leibner, an educator who had for several years studied floating as a tool for helping hyperactive and learning-disabled children, and they quickly merged their talents, building and marketing the first tank designed for home and commercial use: the Samadhi Tank.

By the late 1970s, without any backing by major corporations, without any real interest or publicity in the media, scores of thousands of people had floated, many doing so regularly with tanks in their own homes, or as members of informal tanking networks. Glenn and Lee Perry expanded from simply building tanks to providing commercial tank centers. Gary Higgins of Float to Relax, Inc., came out with a modestly priced home tank and began opening FTR centers all over the United States, with the avowed goal of becoming the "Big Mac" of floating.

In 1978, Paddy Chayefsky published a novel, *Altered States*, based loosely on Lilly's experiences in the float tanks, with a bit of lurid but effective exaggeration. Two years later, a movie based on the book, directed with appropriate bombast and fustian by Ken Russell, was seen by several million people and quickly became a cult classic. The movie, like Chayefsky's book, tells of a scientist who experiments on himself in a floatation tank. Like Lilly, Dr. Eddie Jessup combines floating with powerful psychedelic drugs. Unlike Lilly, Jessup emerges from the tank with a helluva yell and a thick coat of hair, having been transformed into a proto-humanoid ape. The Deep Self indeed!

While the film introduced many to the idea of floating, it also convinced a tremulous few that they would never dare enter a tank for fear they might emerge crazed, filled with an appetite for living beasts. Most people, however, found their curiosity and sense of adventure whetted by the film. Whatever it was that happened in the tank, it sure looked interesting. After the movie's release, the numbers of floaters at public tank centers increased dramatically. And since most who float once want to do it again, many of them bought their own tanks, and sales of tanks went up sharply as well. More publicity came when celebrities like Kris Kristofferson, John Lennon, and Robin Williams acquired float tanks, and athletes took note when the very first year that the Philadelphia Eagles and Philadelphia Phillies installed a float tank in their training room (1980–1981) both teams went on to successful seasons that ended in the Super Bowl and a World Series victory.

Today there are thousands of tanks in everyday use, with commercial float centers in more than a hundred American cities as well as in many European and Japanese cities. While tanks had for many years been used only in the laboratories of university psychology departments, in private homes, or in commercial centers devoted solely to tank use, by 1983 tanks were being used in health spas, biofitness institutes, hospitals, exercise/recreation centers, beauty salons, by professional athletic teams, in corporations, and for "superlearning" courses at several universities.

With the explosion of popular interest in floating, scientific researchers are in the position of struggling to catch up. More and more universities and research facilities have acquired tanks, and in recent months there has been intensified research with tanks in such fields as biochemistry, electromagnetism, brain waves, sleep, behavioral change, suggestibility, reduction of blood pressure, self-regulation, and healing.

The apparatus of today has little in common with the scary air hoses, monster helmets, and complete immersion tanks of twenty years ago. Tank designers have now made available everything from a state of-the-art fully computerized, egg-shaped, luxurious supertank complete with a Jacuzzi-type water massage, an ultraviolet purification system, in-tank lighting, a two-way intercom and underwater stereo that can be controlled by the floater, and optional video screen—a veritable Rolls-Royce of a tank—down through more modest vessels, to simple and inexpensive do-it-yourself home tank kits. Tanks are rapidly losing their air of the exotic, the laboratory, as they become attractive, glossy, high-tech appliances; they are no longer unwieldy curiosity pieces but tools, as accepted and as useful as the home computer.

The comparison with the computer is important. We're told that we have passed from the Industrial Age to the Information Age. Today, information is our strategic resource and real source of power. Information is so essential to life that trend analyst John Naisbitt proposes in his book *Megatrends:* "We need to create a knowledge theory of value to replace Marx's obsolete labor theory of value." [170] He stresses, "In an information society, value is increased by knowledge," and points out that rather than mass-producing cars, our emphasis today is on the mass production of information. Today, says Alvin Toffler, "we still need land and hardware, but the essential property becomes information, and that ... is a revolutionary switch because it's the first form of property that is non-material, non-tangible, and potentially infinite." [251]

The sine qua non of this information age has been the computer. But while the computer is the ideal device for producing, manipulating, and instantaneously communicating information about the social, global reality, and is altering our ways of learning and our modes of entertainment and giving us access to information never before available, its powers are limited when it comes to providing us with information about our inner states, about consciousness, mind, spirit, soul. The float tank, however, offers us direct access to and control over every cell in our bodies, and a wide variety of states of consciousness. What it can give us, then, is *information* about our selves. The tank is thus, in many ways, the computer's internal counterpart, *also* altering our ways of learning and our modes of entertainment, and giving us access to information never before available. So, according to the "knowledge theory of value," the float tank, by increasing our knowledge and information about ourselves, is a truly productive tool—economically, physically, even spiritually, increasing our own value and ability to function effectively in the information society.

Only a decade ago who would have believed that millions of private homes would be supplied with personal computers with 64K of RAM, two disk drives, and more intelligence than the huge room-filling monsters of the sixties? Similarly, it makes sense to think that it won't be too long before millions of homes are equipped with inexpensive float tanks. In fact, the tank seems to be the perfect antidote for the age in which it was created: a technological escape from the pressures of technology, offering stress relief and opportunities for increased self-awareness, creativity, and a rediscovery of and control over the body.

The tank itself is almost too richly symbolic for comfort. Like the computer, it opens to receive the *software* with its unique program — i.e., you—and "runs" the program in an infinity of new ways. Like the space capsule it resembles, it offers escape from the gravitational pull of one reality while speeding you toward another reality as yet unknown. Like that resonant, intriguing phenomenon about which scientists also know very little, the Black Hole, the float tank seems to be like a two-way hatch, offering a way in and a way out at the same time, an opportunity to shrink so small you become infinite, to move so fast you become motionless, to plummet into darkness so deep you emerge in total light.... The metaphoric possibilities are simply too tempting. The only response to such temptation is to relinquish words, at least momentarily, and enter the tank.

PART II

EXPLANATIONS: HOW FLOATATION WORKS

Repose, tranquillity, stillness, inaction—these are the levels of the universe, the ultimate perfection of the Tao.

—CHUANG TZU

In the green water, clear and warm,
Susanna lay.
She searched
The touch of springs
And found
Concealed imaginings.
She sighed,
For so much melody.

—WALLACE STEVENS, **"Peter Quince at the Clavier"**

Tout le malheur des hommes vient d'une seule chose, qui est dèc ne savoir pas demeurer en repos, dans une chambre.

—PASCAL

Tra il dire e il fare c'è de messo il mare.

—OLD ITALIAN SAYING

THREE

DEEP RELAXATION

Paul R. is a young architect whose soft southern drawl seems charmingly out of place in the high-intensity clamor of midtown Manhattan. Recently he shattered his shoulder in a bad skiing accident, and though his orthopedic surgeon was able to set the fracture it continued to cause Paul great pain. It was impossible for him to sleep without pain-killers, and often during the day he would find it hard to concentrate on his work because of the nagging ache. He could ease it with medication, but he didn't like the way the pills made his mind fuzzy. Then he heard from his orthopedic surgeon that floating in an isolation tank could relieve pain, and he was eager to give it a try. When I first met Paul, he'd been floating regularly for several weeks.

"When I first floated it was quite astonishing to me," he mused with a half smile. "I went into the tank with this excruciating pain, and when I came out the pain was gone. I slept that night without any drugs for the first time in weeks! And the next day at work my head was not only clear, I even felt more bouncy and mentally sharp than I *ever* did before I broke my shoulder." He had been floating regularly in the evenings after work, but he felt he was emerging from the tank in such an energetic and creative mood that he was now eager to schedule some early morning pre-work floats, to try to reap the harvest of his increased sense of control, his energy, and the keen pleasure he takes in his work. "And the funny thing is that my doctor says my shoulder is healing by leaps and bounds, much faster now than it was before I started floating. I don't know—you explain it."

Chris, a fashion model in her late twenties, had been the victim of a rape attempt more than two years before she began floating. In fighting off her attacker she had been badly slashed, and while her physical wounds had quickly healed, deeper wounds remained. Frequent attacks of depression would leave her virtually immobilized. Anxiety brought her to the verge of panic several times a week. Though she cared about the man she'd been living with, she was not capable of full sexual response; this, she felt, was one of the reasons the relationship had finally broken apart. Another reason was her dependence on marijuana: The first thing she did every day before getting out of bed was light up a joint, and she stayed high all the time. "I just wanted to stay numb and dumb," she said.

One of her photo assignments included shots of a health club with a floatation tank, and when the photographer went in for a float she decided to take a turn in the tank too. She emerged feeling better than she had in years and decided to explore the process further. She discovered that each float raised her spirits and increased her self-confidence, and that the effect carried over for several days. Her life became more fun and more productive than at any time since the attack. She discovered that she could return to the attack in her mind as she floated, visualizing the scene again and again, replaying it until it seemed to lose its power. "It was like a ghost," she said, "always there, ready to come out and spook me at any time. But now, since I've replayed and revisualized the scene, it's like I've seen through the ghost, and it can't haunt me anymore."

Aram is a criminal lawyer. He uses the tank for a specific purpose: When he's ready to bring a case to trial, he familiarizes himself with all the aspects of the case and then goes into the tank for a long, thoughtful float. In the black silence he allows the various components of the case to circulate in his mind until they begin to fall into place—precedents, strategies, tactics. By the time he comes out of the tank he has a clear sense of what he must do, of how the case will proceed. Similarly, in some complex cases he prepares his summation speech to the jury by going into the tank for a long "rehearsal" float, deciding what he's going to say and visualizing himself going through the speech. The results, he says, have been impressive; he feels more in control of himself, more relaxed, able like a good performer to sense how his act is going over with the audience. The bottom line, he says, is that he is a better lawyer.

Arthur is a midwestern psychologist, intense, very intelligent, somewhat introverted. He is a serious chess player, and he describes his experiences in the float tank with the dispassionate, considered approach he takes toward a game. "I had never been religious," he told me. Raised in a non-religious Jewish family, he had always assumed that spiritual matters were mere excuses for wishful thinking. Middle-aged, he has never been married.

"What brought me to the tank was pure curiosity, nothing else." He explained that it had seemed like something he, as a Ph.D. in psychology with several years of EEG research into sleep, should investigate. "I just wanted to see what would happen," he said. "After about half an hour I began to start thinking about some areas of conflict in the relationship I have with the woman I'm in love with. And as time went on, the areas of conflict seemed to melt away and a sense of harmony took their place. I started to feel as if all problems could be resolved, as if the sense of underlying goodwill between me and this woman could overcome everything."

As he described it, Arthur shook his head in a gesture of disbelief, smiling. "Ultimately it was a type of religious experience. I'm not religious, but if I *were* religious this would be a type of religious experience, a religious revelation: a sense of harmony between me and all other people. The reason I've become very enthusiastic about it is that the feelings I had in the float tank expressed themselves in terms of ideas, which stayed with me. The sense of harmony I imagined having with the woman, whom I had some areas of conflict with—that sense of harmony continued on, and in fact had a positive impact on my relationship with her. Because when I see her now I remember that sense of underlying harmony between me and her, whether or not it exists at the present time, but as a basic state that, if it isn't present now, can easily return."

In the days after that first float, he began to feel the long-term effect. "I often returned to the feelings and ideas I'd had of this religious sense of unity of the universe, harmony, the oneness of the human race. It was an idea that kept coming back to me on frequent occasions."

On his next float Arthur experienced another "religious revelation," and was filled with thoughts about members of his family from whom he'd been alienated for years. Again, he felt a sense of "underlying harmony and unity that I could achieve: a confidence in myself, that if I acted in accordance with the way I am *able* to act, I could achieve a harmony with people with whom I had difficulty being in a harmonious state."

Arthur stressed the long-term effect of the tank experiences: "I would say a permanent impact—it gives me a vision of what life could be like." Now he finds he can recapture the experiences any time he wishes, because they were "strong, vivid." I asked him what he thought was the mechanism of this sudden religious awakening, and he explained: "I would say it's because I was *communicating* with myself in the tank in a way I never did before. It was a unique experience, essentially not comparable to anything else. It's impossible to imagine what a sexual experience is like until you've experienced it—same thing with a float. It's a unique event of its type. Also, in a way it had the same euphoric effect on me that sex does—of feeling a deep sense of harmony with the world, a sense of peacefulness and contentment. Very life affirming.... I plan to keep floating as long as I keep getting these positive results."

Four stories, four orientations: physical body, emotions, intellect, spirit. In truth, these realms cannot be untangled from each other. But they're useful categories for demonstrating an important fact about floating: In each of these realms the tank's effects are clear, immediate, and unmistakable. No one has any doubts that it is the tank's effects, and not something else, that they are feeling. The experience of gravity-free, restricted environmental stimulation *changes* you, and while some of the changes are in the brain, the tank's effects are no more "only in your mind" than are the results of eating a sumptuous dinner when you are very hungry. The changes are real, quantifiable, documented by an impressive amount of rigorous scientific research, controlled studies, statistical analyses of data, not to mention all the ordinary floaters I've spoken to. And in every case I'm aware of, the changes have been beneficial.

Granted, this is quite a claim. There are today numerous techniques people can use that purport to change them for the better, among them running, meditation, biofeedback, psychotherapy, *est*, health spas, at least a million wonderful diets, stop-smoking clinics, Alcoholics Anonymous, Weight Watchers, and more quasi-religious groups and training seminars than you can shake a stick at. The problem with these and scores of other techniques is that they often don't work. Yes, each of them helps many people, but often the success stories are in the minority, while many who have spent hundreds of dollars, or worked hard and disciplined themselves, find that for one reason or another the technique just doesn't seem to work for them. Some lucky people get a runner's high after four or five miles; others just get blisters and tired. Many find they don't have the patience to stick to their meditation long enough to reap all the benefits they've heard about. Some go to this or that seminar only to find that somehow they don't "get it," or if they do, that "it" doesn't seem to help them much.

Floating, however, works for just about everyone (the only exceptions, according to the many doctors, psychologists, psychiatrists, and other health professionals I spoke to, seem to be people with very severe biochemical depression who should see a doctor, and highly obsessive-compulsive people, who will probably have no desire to go into the tank anyway). There is no training required, no secret wisdom, no guru or special decoder ring, no weeks of discipline. In fact, you could probably go into a float tank *determined* that you were going to resist the effects, and you would still emerge changed.

Why is the tank so effective? There are many theories about the mechanisms by which float tanks achieve their results, and today there is an explosion of research into that very question going on in university, hospital, and clinic laboratories around the world. One unmistakable message delivered at the First International Conference on REST and Self-Regulation at Denver, in March 1983, was that we now know more about floating than ever before but we still don't know much, and that there are momentous, potentially revolutionary discoveries to be made. The scientists want more data, larger studies, before they offer conclusive statements. They are wary, knowing that the evidence presented at the convention is startling enough to be susceptible to sensational claims: Manipulate and strengthen your own immune system! Cure sickness! Instant access to the brain's right hemisphere! Dramatic improvements in memory, learning, thinking, creativity! Activate your own pleasure centers! This is, after all, pretty sensational stuff. No one knows quite where it might lead. So for the time being the scientists, full of speculations and wild surmises, devise more studies, more experiments, each approaching the problem from his own direction with his own paradigm or explanation. Their explanations, each of them based on a solid foundation of hard evidence and experimental research, fall into a number of categories which are quite distinct. In the rest of Part II are summaries of the most interesting and important of these explanations. Later in the book, when we look at specific ways the float experience can be put to use in your life, I will refer to—and at times expand upon—these brief summaries.

FOUR

THE ANTI-GRAVITY EXPLANATION

When NASA first put tickets for commercial space-flights on sale, they probably thought the publicity gimmick would be good for a bit of media play. Imagine their surprise when thousands of would-be astronauts actually made reservations. I believe one reason the idea of space-flight is so enticing is that it offers us the only chance we'll ever have, outside our dreams, to experience total weightlessness. Those TV images of our astronauts twirling in black space at the end of a single silver filament, or tumbling in comical free fall across the cabin of their space capsule, are imprinted on our minds. Something in us throbs with excitement to see humans floating weightless: *It's possible* says some inner voice. *It can be done!*

But in real life, gravity seems to be part of the human condition, as inescapable as tooth decay. Like Newton's apple, our bodies ripen, grow heavy, and ultimately fall to earth, though for most of us there is no recumbent pensive genius to observe our fall and derive from it some universal truth.

But just because it is a fact of life does not mean that gravity is the optimal human environment. After all, whatever the mind may be, it is apparently weightless. And for our weightless mind, our too too solid flesh is often like some heavy anchor holding us earthbound when, as our dreams attest, we would really rather be flying, soaring, floating, unencumbered by our ponderous material overcoat.

Up from Gravity: Evolution from Dinosaurs to *Charlie's Angels*

Whatever the driving force behind evolution may be, it has always assumed a single direction for humans: an inexorable progression upward, a continuing struggle to break free from the force of gravity. The fish swam up from the depths, crawled out of the sea; the reptiles slithered on their bellies, evolving *upward*, rising off the earth on legs as they became dinosaurs, turning into winged reptiles and evolving into the creatures we know as birds. Our ancestors, the mammals, also followed their impulses upward, leaving earth and taking up residence in the trees, swinging and tumbling in a sort of free fall from limb to limb. Even today the freedom of the treetops has power over our imagination: Our most potent and evocative lullaby sends babies off to rockabye in the treetop—and when the wind blows the cradle will rock.

But even at the top of the forest our ancestors were still at the mercy of gravity—a single slip, a momentary lapse could mean death. Over millions of years in the high forest we evolved an exquisite awareness of our gravitational orientation, so that even millions of years after our remote ancestors descended from the trees, the fear of falling remains one of the most powerful human instincts, guaranteed to bring children awake in terror from nightmares of plummeting—that ominous awareness that no matter how comforting it is to rock in the treetops, when the bough breaks, that cradle will fall and down will come baby.

So our primate ancestors descended from the trees, not as a retreat from their struggle upward but only to take a different tack, rising from the accustomed four-legged or knuckle-walking posture to become a new creature, *homo erectus*, having made a revolutionary discovery: that you could move along the ground at an incredible speed through a constant nose-thumbing defiance of gravity, repeatedly throwing yourself off balance, in an out-of-control headlong process of falling, breaking the fall with one leg, and instead of recovering balance simply redirecting the energy of the fall. Running! And so the small, timid ape descended from the high forest and became a runner of the savannahs, arguably the greatest runner Earth has ever known, in every headlong stride a defier of gravity—an advancement that most anthropologists believe resulted in our sudden explosive evolution, our development of the huge neocortex, of our complex spoken language, of our ability to fashion and use tools, of our cultivation of social behaviors that still govern our lives today.

In their dreams and myths and rituals these early humans continued to long for escape from gravity, shamans turning into eagles for flights of the spirit, ceremonies directed to the thunderbird, the winged gods, the Chinese flying dragons, Assyrian winged bulls, Egyptian winged deities, the feathered serpent of the Mayans. The Greek gods seemed unaffected by gravity and could transform themselves into swans, if it would help them seduce maidens; Phoebus drove the sun chariot across the heavens; Pegasus, the horse with wings; Hermes with winged sandals. And the Christian heaven is apparently gravity free; when Jesus went there he simply "ascended" from Earth. Of course when the Judeo-Christian angels have to leave the free fall of Paradise and deal with the gravity field of Earth, they use their powerful wings.

Doggedly believing that even unenlightened humans could overcome gravity simply by using their own powers, mad inventors over the centuries developed plans for wings and flying machines. Daedalus, the master craftsman seemed on the right track until Icarus wrecked the equipment. Leonardo kept doodling with plans for his ornithopter, which centuries later became the helicopter. Balloons were the rage of the eighteenth and nineteenth centuries; then came the heavier-than-air flying machines of our century, rockets that could actually escape the planet's gravitational field, satellites, space stations, moon shots, and mad scientists still dreaming of anti-gravity fields and interstellar space ships.

And while humans have not yet been able to free their bodies from gravity for long, one of their greatest evolutionary developments has been their ability to create an entire realm that exists in the gravity-free state: the world of objective knowledge, theoretical systems, scientific learning, philosophy, intellect. Until recently this realm was partially dependent on matter—that part which was preserved in books—and therefore subject to gravity, but now we have invented wonderfully complex tools—radios, televisions, computers—whose effect is to free even the weightless creations of our minds from gravity: *Leave It to Beaver* and *Charlie's Angels* eternal now, beaming outward endlessly into the universe on electromagnetic waves, existing perfectly and without reference to gravity, forever and ever, world without end, floating....

Floating Free from Gravity
Our upright posture is unique and often exhilarating, but gives us, whether we're running, walking, standing, or sitting, a limited area of contact between our bodies and the earth, placing more stress on the body than it was created to withstand. When we're walking or running, for example, all the gravitational pressure of the entire body being jammed against the earth is focused with each step on one relatively small spot, creating thousands of pounds of pressure per square inch. Even simply standing upright causes great gravitational pressure to be exerted on the soles of the feet and the spine. This focusing of large amounts of weight on small parts of the body, and our upright posture, also lead to stress and structural problems in other comparatively weak spots: knee and hip joints, lower back, neck, abdomen. The heart has to work harder than it should to pump the blood upward from the lower body, struggling against gravity. Our bodies try to compensate for the strain of gravity by adopting rigid postures, with the result that we develop chronic muscular tension in certain spots. And with the tension comes pain—lower-back pain, neck pain, tension headache—and a wide range of tension-related problems such as

shallow breathing, high blood pressure, cardiovascular disease, ulcers, asthma.

Gravity is probably the greatest cause of health problems in the United States. The single largest consumer of industrial compensation funds is back trouble, a result of our upright struggle against gravitational force. Gravity even attacks us on a cellular level, and many biologists and gerontologists now feel that the destructive effects of gravity play a significant part in the cell's loss of ability to replicate itself; thus, gravity can be seen as a direct cause of old age and death.

We all know about these aspects of gravity. We're less aware of how insidiously gravity is always on our minds, and in our minds. As we move through our days, much of the brain is kept constantly busy calculating, computing, and dealing with gravity, considering inertia and acceleration, deciding how and where to move what parts of the body to remain upright against the relentless downward pull. It's been estimated that some 90 percent of all the activity affecting our central nervous system is related to gravity, as if some vast computer were incessantly occupied with tedious arithmetical problems, leaving only a small part of it free to run the programs that deal with important questions.

Moshe Feldenkrais concluded that "the bulk of stimuli arriving at the nervous system is from muscular activity constantly affected by gravity," that all our perceptions and sensations take place against this background of muscular activity, and that gravity therefore decreases our sensitivity to and awareness of the external and internal reality. He explains this in terms of the Weber-Fechner Law:

> The general principle at work is as follows. All sensations are related to the stimuli producing them in a fixed manner. For example, if you hold a 20-lb. weight in your hand and you shut your eyes, and if, noiselessly, a certain weight were added on to the weight you already carry, you will not become aware of it unless the additional weight is big enough to produce the least detectable difference in sensation.... In simple words, the Weber-Fechner law means that the smaller the weight you are holding, the smaller is the added or subtracted portion that you will be able to notice.... All sensations in which muscular activity is involved are largely dependent on the smallest amount of tonus persistent in the musculature. When the tonus is the smallest possible, you sense the finest increase in effort. Easy and smooth action is obtained when the aim is achieved by the smallest amount of exertion, which, in turn, is obtained with the minimum tonus present.

The smaller the stimulus present, the smaller is the change that we perceive, or are capable of detecting.... People with a fine kinesthetic sense tend to a low tonic contraction, and are not satisfied until they find the way of doing which involves the smallest amount of exertion; also, the limit to which the unnecessary effort is eliminated is closer to the ideal minimum.[70]

Related to this is our new understanding that learning in the autonomic nervous system is enhanced when all extraneous muscle tension, "background muscle noise," has been turned down as low as possible. Early indications of this came from physiological psychologists Neal Miller and Leo DiCara, who inhibited all muscular activity in rats by injecting them with curare, and found that the paralyzed rats learned much more readily than nonrelaxed rats, mastering such remarkable feats as causing one ear to grow hot while simultaneously making the other ear grow cold.[60,167]

If gravity-related tension reduces our sensitivity and awareness then it seems obvious that reduction of that tension should be beneficial. The floatation tank has this effect: Because of the Epsom salts-saturated water, the human body is completely supported, bobbing on the surface. Feet, legs, hands, arms, spine, head are all supported independently, rather than resting on top of or in a tension relation with one another. Floating does not eliminate gravity, of course. What floating affects, in Lilly's words, is "the peripheral countergravity stimulation exerted by the force of the accelerated mass, i.e., the weight of the body. Floating in water, one distributes this countergravity pressure over the maximum possible area and hence attenuates this source of stimulation to the minimum possible value while still on this planet." [139]

By lowering the gravitational muscular tension, then, we enable ourselves to perceive or detect much smaller sensations, that is, to intensify our sensations. Like DiCara and Miller's curare-dosed rats, we probably could, if we wished, learn to make one ear hot and the other cold, though we might prefer to learn other types of mastery of our autonomic system. By reducing the effects of gravity, the tank seems to have the potential of making us all what sensory deprivation researcher Dr. Ian Wickramsekera of Eastern Virginia Medical School calls "autonomic athletes." [260]

But there are other benefits. Because our bone-muscle system is not constantly straining against gravity, and every muscle can relax more totally than is possible under any other circumstances, we can become intensely aware of knots and hot spots of chronic muscular tension and skeletal strain. No longer hidden or camouflaged by the normal background static of muscular tension, these knots can be pinpointed, consciously attacked, even eliminated, resulting in a euphoric sense of release from the tension that psychiatrist Wilhelm Reich called our "body armor."

The release from gravity also allows the blood to circulate more freely and completely, reaching parts of the body that may be unhealthy because of cardiovascular constriction (caused by things like smoking, cholesterol clogging, and tension), and in the process allowing the heart to operate more efficiently with less effort. Another result is a drop in blood pressure. The pulse rate slows. By relieving gravitational pressure on joints, tendons, ligaments, bones, and muscles, the tank alleviates temporarily the chronic pain of such ailments as bursitis, arthritis, tendinitis, and traumatic or structural pains from bruises, sprains, broken bones, and muscle strain. It's likely that Paul the architect experienced relief from the pain of his broken shoulder in part because of the tank's anti-gravity effect. Not only did floating eliminate the downward pull on the shattered bone, but by alleviating the tension in the rest of his body it probably increased the flow of blood to the injured area, and along with the blood the flow of biochemicals that could promote the rapid healing noted by his doctor.

In addition to a stronger flow of blood to every part of the brain, there is a freeing of those parts of the brain usually devoted to computing and dealing with the effects of gravity on the body. In a very true sense, floating allows us to put the brain to use dealing with matters of the mind and spirit.

One of the most common responses to the float experience is a feeling of coming home, to a familiar place. Some have explained this as an experience of return to the womb. But I think it goes even deeper, to a cellular, perhaps precellular level, to sensations that are native to our collective unconscious. The exhilaration we feel in the tank is something imprinted in our genes, something we have always known, always longed for: the release from gravity, the escape from the body, the freedom from the pull of the cells—that is, Floating.

FIVE

THE BRAIN WAVE EXPLANATION

By now few are unaware that the activity of the human brain creates patterns of electrical energy, that the electrical signals of the brain can be monitored by placing electrodes against the scalp, and that a device known as an electroencephalograph (or EEG) can record the brain waves by means of a sensitive mechanical pen tracing, across a long sheet of paper, a mountain range of jagged lines—as immortalized in a thousand science fiction movies and television hospital series. Flat line equals brain death—cart him away, nurse. These brain signals have a tendency to fall into certain patterns which scientists have classified in four types:

Beta. When the brain is generating mostly beta waves, whose frequency is about 13-30 Hz (that is, a rhythm of 13 to 30 cycles per second), it is in what is called its waking rhythm: The brain is focusing on the world outside itself, or dealing with concrete, specific problems.

Alpha. As the brain waves slow down they take on a more coherent rhythm, and can be seen on the EEG as a regular sawtooth pattern at about 8-12 Hz. These waves are often present when the brain is alert but unfocused, and most people generate alpha waves when their eyes are closed, even if only in bursts of one or two seconds. Frequently, alpha waves are associated with feelings of relaxation and calmness.

Theta. As calmness and relaxation deepen into drowsiness, the brain shifts to slower, more powerfully rhythmic waves with a frequency of about 4-7 Hz. Everyone generates these theta waves at least twice per day: in those fleeting instants when we drift from conscious drowsiness into sleep, and again when we rise from sleep to consciousness as we awaken. The theta state is accompanied by unexpected, unpredictable, dreamlike but very vivid mental images (known as *hypnagogic* images). Often these startlingly real images are accompanied by intense memories, particularly childhood memories. Theta offers access to unconscious material, reverie, free association, sudden insight, creative inspiration. It is a mysterious, elusive state, potentially highly productive and enlightening, but experimenters have had a difficult time studying it, and it is hard to maintain, since people tend to fall asleep as soon as they begin generating large amounts of theta.

Delta.   Cycling at an extremely slow frequency (.5-4 Hz), delta rhythms are produced when people are deeply asleep or otherwise unconscious.

Throughout the 1960s, experimenters discovered that with the use of equipment that electrically monitored selected physical functions, humans could learn to generate those functions at will. While biofeedback equipment could be made to monitor just about any physical function, researchers often focused on the production of alpha waves. Stress was a problem shared by almost everyone, and an accepted antidote to stress was relaxation; since alpha waves accompanied relaxation, and were relatively easy to learn to produce at will, clinical biofeedback experts assumed that if you could learn to generate alpha waves, you would automatically become relaxed. In the early 1970s, with the advent of relatively inexpensive equipment came an explosion of interest in biofeedback, and *alpha* became the catchword seized on by the mass media and seekers of expanded consciousness.

Almost unnoticed amidst the hoopla surrounding alpha was an earlier study by Akira Kasamatsu and Tomio Hirai which analyzed EEG tests of Zen monks going into deep meditative states. The study showed that as the monks went into meditation they passed through four stages: the appearance of alpha waves, an increase of alpha amplitude, a decrease of alpha frequency, and finally (for those with the most skill at meditation), the production of long trains of theta waves. Interestingly, the four states "were parallel with the disciples' mental states, which were evaluated by a Zen master, and disciples' years spent in Zen training." In other words, the more meditative experience a monk had, the more theta he generated (i.e., those monks who had more than twenty years of experience generated the greatest amounts of theta waves). And, even in the depths of theta, the monks were not asleep but mentally alert.

Elmer and Alyce Green, biofeedback researchers at the Menninger Clinic, became interested in the theta state (they'd been studying the brain waves of Swami Rama when he told them: "Alpha is nothing!") and began training subjects to generate theta waves consciously. They found theta "to be associated with a deeply internalized state and with a quieting of the body, emotions, and thoughts, thus allowing usually 'unheard or unseen things' to come to consciousness in the form of hypnagogic imagery." As their theta training groups progressed, they were surprised to find a "high frequency of subject reports indicating *integrative* experiences leading to feelings of psychological well-being." Many of the subjects began reporting spontaneous improvements in personal relationships. Many vivid memories of long-forgotten childhood events arose: "They were not like going through a memory in one's mind but rather like an experience, a reliving." Subjects reported both physical and psychological well-being, and the Greens discovered that people with the most hypnagogic imagery were "psychologically healthier, had more social poise, were less rigid and conforming, and were more self-accepting and creative" than those who produce little or no hypnagogic imagery.

The Greens were surprised by their findings, and concluded that the theta state caused people to "experience a new kind of body consciousness very much related to their total well-being." Physiologically, the theta state seemed to bring "physical healing, physical regeneration." In the emotional domain, the theta state was "manifested in improved relationships with other people as well as greater tolerance, understanding, and love of oneself and of one's world." In the mental domain, theta ability involves "new and valid ideas or syntheses of ideas, not primarily by deduction, but springing by intuition from unconscious sources."

Understandably excited by the extraordinarily beneficial powers of the ability to generate theta waves, the Greens undertook a research project they called Brain-wave Training for Mental Health, to train psychotherapists to assist their clients in learning the technique. The problem is that it is not easy to learn to produce theta waves; first of all, theta usually leads to sleep. And as the Greens point out, "In order to produce theta consciously it is necessary to have a quiet body, tranquil emotions, and quiet thoughts *all at the same time*."[87] Some cynics might retort that if one had a quiet body, tranquil emotions, and quiet thoughts, one would have no need for any training. The fact is, few people know how to achieve this happy simultaneity, and few have the necessary discipline and patience to learn. After all, it seems to take Zen monks some twenty years to be able to generate this state at will.

But as anyone who has floated is aware, the quiet body, tranquil emotions, and quiet thoughts formula is a perfect description of the floater's circumstances. Could it be that floating increases and facilitates the production of theta waves? Research indicates that this is indeed so. As early as 1956, John Lilly was noting that the state of mind in the float tank was "hypnagogic," full of "reveries and fantasies," with much visual imagery and many child-hood memories, and mental events that were "surprising to the ego"—all characteristics of theta activity. J.P. Zubek, investigating "EEG changes in perceptual and sensory deprivation," reported that theta waves became prominent. A recent study by Gary S. Stern, associate professor of psychology at the University of Colorado at Denver, found that "the significant effect of floating ... indicates that individuals who had floated in the isolation tank for one hour significantly raised their theta level." [229]

A large controlled study by Professor Thomas E. Taylor, of Texas A & M, analyzed the effects of floating on several types of learning abilities, compar-ing floaters with people in a relaxed state in a dark, quiet room. Both the float and non-float groups were measured with EEGs, and the study found that floating leads to an increase in the generation of theta waves. [247]

Biofeedback expert Thomas Budzynski, clinical director of the Biofeedback Institute of Denver and professor of psychiatry at the University of Colorado Medical Center, is currently doing research involving the meas-urement by EEG of the brain during hypnosis. He has concluded that float tanks increase the production of theta waves, and believes that this has great potential for opening the mind to learning: "We take advantage of the fact that the hypnagogic state, the twilight state, between waking and sleep, has these properties of uncritical acceptance of verbal material, or almost any material it can process. What if you could cause a person to sustain that state, and not fall asleep? I believe floatation tanks are an ideal medium for doing that." [38]

Budzynski's observation that the tank is ideal for maintaining wakeful-ness while in theta is supported by almost everyone who has done work in the area of sensory deprivation. Jay Shurley and John Lilly were probably the first to point out that the tank facilitates wakefulness in most users. Others (A.M. Ross, and colleagues, for instance) have since indicated various reasons for this, such as the body's natural homeostatic mechanism to maintain alert-ness, the "sensoristat," which creates a unique combination of high brain arousal and low muscular arousal. It's important to emphasize this point: Usually when you enter the theta state you fall asleep, but the tank causes the floater to generate large amounts of theta, yet remain awake. This means that the vivid hypnagogic imagery, the creative ideas, the *eureka* moments and light bulb thoughts, the "knowing" feeling, the "integrative experiences" mentioned by Elmer and Alyce Green, with all the resultant beneficial effects on body, emotions, and mind, are available to the floater; in the tank these experiences come while the floater remains awake, so they remain a part of the floater's conscious mind even after he has emerged.

Arthur, the psychologist who had a "religious revelation" while floating, said, "The reason I've become very enthusiastic about it is that the feelings I had in the float tank expressed themselves in terms of ideas *which stayed with me.*" When he tried to explain this extraordinary experience, Arthur said, "I went into such deep relaxation that I felt a very special form of communication with myself. I was communicating with thoughts and feelings I normally disregard." And finally he pointed out that the floats had a permanent impact on him: He is able to recapture the experiences at any time he wishes, because they were so "strong" and "vivid." It is evident that Arthur experienced the vivid hypnagogic imagery so characteristic of theta, and because of the tank's uncommon ability to maintain a floater's wakefulness in the theta state, he was able to remember clearly everything he felt there. When Arthur describes the permanent impact the experiences have had on his life, he seems to be a walking example of the increased psychological well-being researchers have found to be characteristic of theta.

It's intriguing to note that theta activity is prominent in young children. Kenneth Pelletier notes: "As children develop, [theta] rhythms decline proportionately as alpha activity increases until the age of ten or eleven, when the normal adult EEG pattern of beta dominance becomes established."[187] Those who remember their childhood, or who have children of their own, will immediately recognize the theta states of childhood, when children can become so engrossed in an activity they seem to lose contact with the external world. Studies have shown that many experiences are "state bound," that is, they can only be relived fully when we reenter the mind-set of our first encounter with them. That being true, it makes sense that when we reenter the theta state so common to childhood (yet so rare in normal adult life), childhood events return with astonishing clarity. Also linking theta waves to memory, a study of the learning process in rats indicates that theta waves seem to signal the brain's readiness to process memories. This memory-enhancing or memory-liberating quality of theta, offering freer access to one's past, is one reason why many psychotherapists are finding float tanks an invaluable adjunct to therapy, assisting and accelerating the process of self-exploration.

The Greens and other researchers have remarked that many great creative discoveries have resulted from hypnagogic imagery experienced in a theta state. The chemist Friedrich Kekule, for example, vividly described his state of "reverie" in which he suddenly saw a mental image of atoms forming a chain, and of snakes biting their tails; his subsequent discovery that organic compounds occur in closed rings has been described as "the most brilliant piece of prediction to be found in the whole range of organic chemistry."[136] There are countless stories of such moments of inspiration and creativity occurring when the thinker is nodding off to sleep, or gazing into the sky, or wandering lonely as a cloud. Virtually all of them speak of the drowsiness, the physical relaxation, the vivid imagery appearing unexpectedly, that mark them as examples of the theta state. The tank cannot make geniuses of us all, but its ability to put us into a theta state suggests that it can be a valuable aid in promoting creativity.

SIX

THE LEFT-BRAIN
RIGHT-BRAIN EXPLANATION

The human brain, removed from its protective shell, the skull, looks something like a large walnut half, deeply fissured and split into two parts by a deep central crevasse. These two parts of the brain, known as hemispheres or lobes, are connected only by thick bundles of nerves. Through observation of the effects of head wounds, humans have known for thousands of years that damage to the left side of the brain has different effects on the injured person's mental and physical capacities than damage to the right side of the brain. Then, in a series of extraordinary studies during the 1960s, brain researchers Roger Sperry, Michael Gazzaniga, Joseph Bogen, and others studied the brains and capabilities of patients who had undergone radical surgery that totally separated the two hemispheres by severing the *corpus callosum*, the thick band of nerve fibers connecting them. These now historic studies caused excitement and astonishment by demonstrating that not only does each hemisphere of the cortex have its own train of conscious thought and its own memories, but that the two sides *think or operate in fundamentally different modes*.

Left Brain. As research progressed, evidence piled up that the brain is "crosswired" to the body—with the right hemisphere controlling the left half of the body, and the left hemisphere controlling the right half and that for the majority of people the left hemisphere is dominant. This left brain seems to think analytically, sequentially, logically, with an orientation in time.

Right Brain. The right brain, on the other hand, tends to process information in a mostly nonverbal, simultaneous, intuitive, nonlinear, timeless, imagistic manner. It seems to be the seat of those flashes of insight that have been called the Eureka event.

A recent study by brain researcher Justin Sergent, of McGill University, has challenged this familiar theory of hemispheric function; the study proposes that the left hemisphere excels at *detail*, processing in formation that is small-scale, requiring fine resolution, while the right hemisphere is best at pattern recognition and large-scale, non-detailed processing.[43] The right brain is by nature a good guesser, rapidly absorbing information in broad outline, while the left hemisphere must take its time and deal with details. Although this new research questions certain assumptions of the usual right/left paradigm, it actually reaffirms the essential differences in function between the two hemispheres: In a sense, the right hemisphere supplies the shape and the frame, while the left fills in the details.

Sinister Thoughts, Subversion from the Left

As research into brain lateralization progressed and scientists began to understand how the dominance of one or the other hemisphere could not only color one's perceptions of external reality but actually determine the reality one perceived, it became clear that our culture valued and cultivated those qualities associated with left-brain activity more than it did those of the right brain. Many have noted, for example, that even the word *right* has positive connotations beyond those of physical position: The very concept of "rightness" as that which is correct, upright, fit, convenient, free from guilt, is opposed by the concept of leftness, with its connotations of evil (the Latin word for left is *sinister*). Probably the most stunning demonstration of how completely oriented toward the left brain our culture is, is the fact that surgeons have removed the entire right hemisphere from conscious patients *without their noticing the slightest st change tit awareness.*

Left-hemisphere dominance is powerfully reinforced by our educational system. When we're born the two hemispheres seem to work independently but with equal powers. In their play, their fantasies, their thinking, children show strong right-brain activity—they're diffuse, intuitive, visual, musical, and they seem to have no sense of time, responding to unpredictable inner rhythms. But in the primary and secondary schools, these right-brain qualities are causes for criticism or even punishment. Fantasizing is not welcome in the classroom, teachers are not usually receptive to intuitive answers to questions, and in every classroom there is a large clock on the wall. Students who won't curb their right brains are seen as day dreamer, dawdlers, lazy, disruptive.

By the time students reach college, left-hemisphere dominance is firmly established. Skill at using the verbal, analytic hemisphere is rewarded by good grades. Yet in one experiment, college students were tested in their intuitive thinking ability, and when the results were compared to the students' grade point average, there was almost no correlation at all; the study concluded that "intuitive thinking is clearly *unrelated to college grades.*" [259]

While left-brain skills are rewarded by good grades, and are highly valued by our culture, they are not sufficient for complete functioning and a fully rewarding life. In fact, most productive thinkers and *all* recognized geniuses have insisted that their ideas and creative energies have flowed from that deep pool of wisdom that has been called the unconscious. Logic, words, and details are important, but they are only tools; they are not reality themselves, but useful symbols or means of approaching reality. To be effectively used, they need the intuitive, large-scale, synthesis-making abilities of the right hemisphere.

In recent years many have recognized the dangers of left-hemisphere dominance and have undertaken in various ways to emphasize the right-brain functions. Meditation, yoga, Zen, consciousness-altering drugs, chanting, dancing, running, guided dreaming, visualization, self-hypnosis, and many other techniques have been used to open up the right hemisphere. But all the evidence now available suggests there is no more reliable and efficient way for a human to gain access to the contents of the right hemisphere than by entering a float tank for an hour or so.

Research into the brain waves of the two hemispheres of floaters indicates that floating increases right-brain function. Thomas Budzynski, who is engaged in EEG measurement of the hemispheres under varying conditions, made it clear in a speech he delivered at the Denver REST conference. "In a float condition," he said, "left-hemisphere faculties are somewhat suspended and the right hemisphere ascends in dominance." [38]

While an increasing amount of research evidence demonstrates that floating has this effect of opening up the right hemisphere, anecdotal evidence is just as impressive. Of the scores of people I have talked with about floating, *every one of them* has mentioned some incidence of sudden awareness of right-brain activity. Paul, the young architect with the broken shoulder who went into the tank to ease his pain, was surprised to note an increased ability to visualize architectural details, solve problems, and create with an originality surpassing anything he had been capable of before. Chris, the fashion model who'd never been able to talk herself out of her anxiety, rid herself of it by using the images that flowed from the nonverbal right hemisphere. Arthur, the scholarly Ph.D. who had always gotten high grades but had never been able to form a satisfactory relationship with a woman, fascinated with details but scornful of religion—surely a left-brain-dominant person—suddenly found himself filled with a deep sense of wholeness, harmony, and a new vision of how to love. It was, he said, "a totally new kind of communication with myself." The communication was with his previously inhibited right hemisphere and its ability to see things in a large-scale, unified way.

How does the tank accomplish so easily what many must work and train for in rigorous meditative techniques? To use the day-night metaphor, in the sunshine of the day it is impossible to see the faint bits of light scattered through the sky by the millions. Just so are the diffuse, subtle contents of the right hemisphere drowned out and overpowered by the noisy chattering of the verbal/analytical hemisphere. Floatation, by turning off the external stimuli, plunges us into a literal and figurative darkness, where suddenly the entire universe of stars and galaxies is spread out before our eyes.

Floating enables left-dominant people to gain access to the right brain more readily than other techniques do because the other methods seek to make people experience something whose location is still a mystery to them—like telling someone to look very hard for stars at high noon of a sunny day. People have developed such powerful strategies to maintain left-brain dominance that they simply refuse to relinquish them. The chatter never stops; the sun of consciousness never sets. Even the thought of nightfall fills them with a deep dread—at night the wild beasts prowl.

In the tank, on the other hand, there is no struggle to guide the left-oriented person toward some ill-defined right-brain awareness. You close the door, the light goes out, the chatter stops, and there it is.

Two Halves Make a Whole: Hemispheric Integration

Despite the immense importance, even necessity, of being open to the large-scale, creative, unifying vision of the right hemisphere, it would be a mistake to think that right-brain thinking is somehow "better" or on a higher moral plane than left-brain thought. Many who have correctly perceived the importance of the nonverbal hemisphere, and have realized the damage done to our culture and our world by left-brain dominance, make the error of viewing right-brain dominance as a noble goal. "Look where logical, analytical, verbal thinking has gotten us," they seem to say. "Our only hope is the right hemisphere! All power to the right brain!" They then plunge into the dark depths of the unconscious.

To call those depths dark is no mere figure of speech. Neurologist Marcel Kinsbourne points out that the different hemispheres are not only specialized for mental processes but also that "it is now becoming increasingly clear that each hemisphere also supports a different emotional state.

Neuropsychologists in several countries have found evidence that the right hemisphere is involved in negative feelings and their expression, while the left is associated with positive feelings and their expression." Citing split-brain studies, Kinsbourne asserts that "the left hemisphere of the split-brain person seems to be innocent of evil."[129]

One brain researcher has shown films to experimental volunteers through special lenses that allow the films to be seen by the right or left hemisphere only; the experiments showed, says Carl Sagan, "a remarkable tendency for the right hemisphere to view the world as more unpleasant, hostile, and even disgusting than the left hemisphere.... The negativism of the right hemisphere is apparently strongly tempered in everyday life by the more easygoing left hemisphere. But a dark and suspicious emotion tone seems to lurk in the right hemisphere, which may explain some of the antipathy felt by our left hemisphere selves to the 'sinister' quality of the left hand and the right hemisphere." [204]

An explanation for this may lie in the fact that, as noted, the right hemisphere deals with information on a broad scale, tending to perceive things as shapes and patterns. However, seeing patterns and unity in external reality is a characteristic of what we call paranoia. There's no way we can know whether the patterns our right hemisphere discerns are real or imagined unless we submit them to the more detailed evaluation of our left hemisphere. On the other hand, as Sagan points out, "Mere critical thinking, without creative and intuitive insights, without the search for new patterns, is sterile and doomed. To solve complex problems in changing circumstances requires the activity of both cerebral hemispheres."

McGill researcher Justin Sergent, who contends that the left brain specializes in detailed processing, the right in pattern recognition and large-scale processing, concludes: "This points to a cooperation between hemispheres whose respective limitations and predispositions allow for complementary capacities in processing information." [43]

While we've known of the lateralization of the brain's functions for only a few years, the dangers of the imbalance of the two brains, of what Charles Hampden-Turner calls the "pathology of splitting,"[94] have been known to us for millennia. The perception of the harm done by the incapacity of the two lobes to harmonize and integrate was probably one of our species' earliest and clearest, and certainly remains one of its most deeply felt, symbolized in such potent myths as the Fall of Man, the rending of the Veil of the Temple, the shadow self or the double or doppelgänger, and in the "splitting" of schizophrenia, the antagonism between male and female, the existence of God and Devil, and so on.

The remedy for this dangerous internal division has also been known for millennia; virtually every religion, philosophy, psychology, and healing practice has stressed that the road to ultimate wisdom and health lies through a balancing and harmonizing of the functions of the hemispheres, symbolized variously as the unity of yin and yang, day and night, mind and body, consciousness and unconscious, ego and id, creative and receptive, heaven and earth, male and female, inner and outer, self and others—seen not as oppositions but rather as complementary parts of a single whole, brought into proper relation, which can be called symmetry, dialectic, harmony, resonance, congruence, dialogue.

Although techniques for attaining this harmony have been taught as long as there have been humans, it has often been assumed that the concept of symmetry was merely the metaphor. While this may be partially true, we're now discovering that the ideas of symmetry and integration are also true in the most literal and concrete way. Various experimenters have used a variety of equipment, including the EEG and the PET scan (positron emission tomography, in which a radioactive isotope injected into the bloodstream is carried to areas of high metabolism—e.g., the brain—so that a picture can be taken), to measure the activity of the two hemispheres while the subject is in various emotional states and performing various mental functions. Their conclusions have been clear:

≈ British psychologist C. Maxwell Cade, recording electroencephalograms of more than four thousand people, discovered that "all the unusual abilities that some people are able to manifest (self-control of pain and healing, healing of others, telepathy, etc.) are associated with changes in the EEG pattern toward a more bilaterally symmetrical and integrated form." [40]

≈ Dr. Bernard Glueck, director of research at the Hartford Institute of Living, conducted extensive tests on large numbers of meditators, and found that the EEG patterns of successful meditators showed an increased synchrony between the left and right hemispheres; that is, both sides functioned together, in harmony. [84]

≈ Neurologist J. P. Banquet also did EEG studies of meditators, and provided push buttons so that the subjects could signal when they were entering different levels or stages of meditation. Banquet noticed that when meditators signaled they were in "deep meditation" or "pure awareness," their brain waves had become *in phase*, and *synchronized* in both hemispheres of the brain, a condition Banquet called *hypersynchrony*. He concluded that this harmony of hemispheres is the single most outstanding EEG characteristic of "deep" states of consciousness.[10,11]

Such findings have led writer Peter Russell, author of *The Brain Book*, to conclude: "As a species we seem to be moving in the direction of greater communication between the two halves. A similar phenomenon seems to be happening at the level of individual evolution, personal development of awareness resulting in an increased communication between the hemispheres.[203]

This evolutionary step forward means we're learning to use our brains more efficiently. The specialization in function of the separate hemispheres, in fact, has the value of increasing our brain capacity. Each hemisphere analyzes the input in its own style, and only then exchanges information with the other half, after much initial processing and sorting is already completed. Budzynski, along with other brain researchers, has compared this to having two separate computers in our heads. We are thus "able to run two programs on everything that happens to us," he says, "and then choose the best one. That's where we have the big jump on lower animals." By our access to two simultaneous streams of information which we can compare and integrate, we are made simply more intelligent. Research is now, underway to measure the brain waves of both hemispheres while the subject is in the tank, using a waterproof "electrode cap," but preliminary studies (EEGs made of floaters who have just emerged from the tank) indicate that this synchronization and balancing of hemispheres does take place during floatation.

Synchronization of brain waves, hemispheric harmony, is one explanation for the great increase in productivity, performance, and efficiency, and the generalized feelings of competence, confidence, and wholeness experienced by floaters. Recall, for example, Arthur's "special sort of communication" with himself, which resulted in "a feeling of unity of all things, harmony, wholeness." The tank does not block or inhibit the left hemisphere, but simply changes its role from one of dominance to one of partnership with the other hemisphere, enabling floaters to use all their mental powers.

SEVEN

THE THREE-BRAIN
EXPLANATION

Billy is a painter who has recently begun floating. He and I have been friends for almost fifteen years, so when I describe him as an easygoing and enormously peaceable fellow, I speak from long experience. A recent conversation swung around to floating, and I asked him how it had affected him. It made him very mellow, he said. Any interesting experiences? I asked. No, said Billy. Oh well, there was this one thing.... A few days before, he'd just gotten out of the tank and come home. "As usual, I felt laid back. I was down on the floor playing with Dan [his young son], when the boy from downstairs came up yelling, 'Why's he hitting my mother?' I went out to find this junkie from downstairs punching out his mother, a sixty-three-year-old woman. You know how hard it is to get me mad. I *never* get in fights, right? But this time there was no hesitation. I just jumped over the banister and blindsided him, coldcocked him, beat his head on the floor, until I heard him screaming and stopped. The guy was looking at me with a strange expression, saying, 'Man, you're crazy.' I just acted, pure action, no thinking or wondering what to do. When the cops came to take him away my first thought was: *What a way to waste a float!* I wanted to run out and grab the guy and say, 'Give me twenty dollars so I can go do another float!' I really creamed the guy," Billy said, shaking his head in disbelief. "I don't know what got into me."

What got into him is interesting, and it has to do with a horse and a crocodile.

Lying Down with the Crocodile and Horse

While the split between the right and left hemispheres is much discussed these days, it can be argued that the most dangerous division in the human brain is not the lateral but the vertical. This is an idea convincingly argued by Paul D. MacLean, chief of the Laboratory of Brain Evolution and Behavior at the National Institutes of Mental Health. MacLean's "triune brain theory" identifies three separate physiological levels of the human brain, each corresponding with a stage in our evolutionary history.[156]

The most ancient part of the brain—that is, the one that evolved first—is a combination of the spinal cord, the brain stem, and the midbrain. This system, which controls basic self-preservative, reproductive and life-sustaining functions, such as respiration, heart regulation, and blood circulation, is pretty much now what it has been for millions of years; the same primitive brain was present in the most ancient reptiles, as it is in reptiles today. This part of the human brain makes us all brother to dragons, and therefore MacLean has called it the *reptile brain*.

The next part of the brain to develop is known as the *limbic system*, which is situated atop the reptile brain in somewhat the manner of a hand clutching the knob of a cane. Because we share this area of the brain with other mammals, such as the rabbit, rat, and horse, it has been called the old mammal or *paleomammalian brain*.

The last area of the brain to develop is the *neocortex*, the mass of convoluted gray matter that overlies and surrounds the core of the older two brains. This brain is the one that is divided into left and right hemispheres, and connected by the *corpus callosum*. It is the neocortex that truly distinguishes humans from other animals. "Speaking allegorically of these three brains within a brain," MacLean has written, "we might imagine that when the psychiatrist bids the patient to lie on the couch, he is asking him to stretch out alongside a horse and a crocodile. The crocodile may be willing and ready to shed a tear and the horse to neigh and whinny, but when they are encouraged to express their troubles in words, it soon becomes evident that their inability is beyond the help of language training. Little wonder that the patient who has personal responsibility for these animals and who must serve as their mouthpiece is sometimes accused of being full of resistances and reluctant to talk." [154]

The Reptile Brain   is, as the name implies, that part of the human brain that coldly watches and waits, stays alert or nods off to sleep. It is the location of the reticular activating system (RAS), the "alarm bell of the brain," which determines our arousal level and our state of awareness and attention. The RAS distinguishes between events that are normal and those that are out of the ordinary, and makes sure we pay attention to the new while allowing us to ignore the familiar. A mother can sleep through a raging storm but awaken to a whimper from her baby because of the arousing, attention-directing function of the RAS; for this reason it has been called the "volume control knob" of the brain.

The RAS not only arouses us and focuses our attention, it can also inhibit brain function, causing us to fall asleep or lapse into coma. And by regulating the amount of external stimulation it will permit to reach the other parts of the brain, the RAS plays a crucial role in determining how outgoing and sociable, or indrawn and shy, we are. Like a filter, the RAS lets through only certain information, and a certain amount of information, to our awareness. People whose reticular activating systems filter out a great deal must give themselves lots of stimulation to feel alive; they will be known as extroverts. A person whose RAS is quite open, admitting large quantities of material to awareness, will not need to seek out additional stimulation and will be known as an introvert.

Many a person whose RAS keeps him or her open to stimulation will find the level of arousal too high for comfort, and will turn down the volume control by drinking alcohol or taking other depressant drugs, which does indeed cause the RAS to lower the stimulation but which can also depress other functions of the reptile system, such as respiration—which is why drug overdoses can cause death. Another person who wants to force *more* stimulation through the filter of the RAS may take stimulants, or speed. Floating in an isolation tank has a powerful effect on the RAS, causing it to put the floater into a deeply relaxed yet highly alert state of calm reverie. Thus, it makes sense that floating should have a strong effect on such things as alcohol and drug consumption, neurotic behavior, shyness, introversion and extroversion, aesthetic and spiritual awareness.

The Paleomammalian Brain, or the horse brain, is the control center for another approach to life: the emotions. Here are generated all our vivid emotions and states of mind: rage, fear, panic, pleasure, bliss. Electrical stimulation of the limbic system can cause sudden frenzy, terror, symptoms similar to psychotic states or psychedelic drug induced states—and in fact most psychedelic substances act by influencing this part of the brain. Messages received from the environment pass through here on their way to the neocortex, and the paleomammalian brain's mood-altering capabilities can color these messages, affecting our emotional spectrum so that we see the world through rose-colored glasses or in a blue funk, despite the intention of our neocortex to view things Not surprisingly, then, this is the area in which such responses as affection, sexual behavior, parental attachment, altruistic impulses, and even love originate.

These moods and emotions are in many ways inseparable from physiological responses in the autonomic nervous system—the dilating blood vessels that make us blush, or flush with anger; the pounding heart that signifies passion or terror. Love can make our hearts go pit-apat and fill us with ecstasy, but the artificial stimulation of a certain part of the limbic brain with a very slight electrical current can have the same result. During brain surgery, doctors can touch parts of the limbic system with electrodes and cause the patient to feel rage, depression, joy, panic. "It would seem," wrote MacLean, "that the raw stuff of emotion is built into the circuitry of the brain."[104] In ways that are still not completely clear, there is a link between emotions (which are immaterial) and the body (which is matter), between thought and physiology, between external conditions and internal states, between voluntary and involuntary muscles. The link must be a sort of alchemical philosophers' stone, able to transmute thought into action, stimulus into emotion, spirit into matter—and vice versa. This mysterious link, or coordinating center, is the limbic system, called the *visceral brain* by MacLean for its control over the body's viscera, or internal organs.

Ruling the limbic system is the *hypothalamus*. Known as "the brain's brain," this structure is the main regulator of all bodily functions, the most powerful of the brain's emotion-causing centers, controlling those innate biological drives and processes most fundamental to survival (such as hunger, thirst, sex, maintaining body temperature) and exercising a pervasive influence over all our emotions and drives. It is in the hypothalamus that electrical stimulation causes intense pleasure; there are areas known as pleasure centers and pleasure pathways. The hypothalamus also is the key regulator of our response to pain and stress. All sensory information from the outside world is delivered to the hypothalamus; if the information is interpreted as stressful, the hypothalamus releases neurochemicals that cause glands such as the pituitary and adrenals to release stimulating chemicals into the bloodstream, resulting in the "adrenaline rush" known as the fight-or-flight response. In a sense, then, the hypothalamus is the main agent of transmutation, changing sensory information from the outside world into neurochemicals that produce profound physical and emotional changes.

Clearly, anything that influences the hypothalamus will alter the entire mind/body system. So it is most interesting that recent studies by endocrinologists and other scientists show that floating has a direct and very substantial influence on the hypothalamus. Because of its powerful, rapid, and long-lasting influence on the limbic system, floating has an enormous effect on mood, emotions, control over autonomic functions, and all aspects of the mind-body interrelationship.

The Neocortex is the convoluted mass of gray matter that covers these older brains like a thick ball of cotton at the tip of a cotton swab. This "thinking cap" accompanied and in part caused that stunning burst of evolution that produced the unique thinking primate known as *Homo sapiens*—a burst of brain growth so fast that many experts speak of it as a brain "explosion."

This "roof brain" is the seat of our high-order abstract, cognitive functions: memory, judgment, intellect. Here we receive and process visual and auditory perceptions; here we're able to remember the past, to anticipate and in a sense to shape the future. Here we create and manipulate what is perhaps the greatest human talent, language. And, while the older brains possess intimate (but unconscious) connections with the autonomic nervous system, the neocortex is the place where our *conscious* thinking is done. It is in charge of our voluntary movements and actions.

According to MacLean's triune brain theory, these three separate brains are superimposed on one another, so that while many of their functions overlap, they are all quite different in chemistry, in structure, in action, in style. It's almost as if the force of evolution, having experimented with one type of brain and found it wanting, decided to try another approach entirely, then another, without going back and eliminating or significantly modifying the earlier versions. Each of the three brains, says MacLean, has its own drives, its own memory, its own problem solving ability; each functions as a fairly autonomous brain on its own level.

The Wild Horses of Schizophysiology

Well, aren't three brains better than one? The cortex's two lateral hemispheres, operating like two separate computers, add to the power and "intelligence" at our command. Perhaps our three vertical brains could also increase our potential fitness to survive.

This could well be so, if in fact the three brains worked together harmoniously. Unfortunately, this is not the case. As MacLean points out, the human brain is hindered by a ruinous "design error"; there is insufficient communication and coordination between the "rational" neocortex and the two older levels of the brain. In that failing, not in the lateral division of the brain into right and left hemisphere, is the origin of our lethal split between reason and emotion, higher and lower selves.

The split between the two hemispheres is bridged effectively by the *corpus callosum*, and while our culture has allowed one hemisphere to gain dominance, the two halves *can* be fully integrated and synchronized. However, MacLean stresses that there is no such means of effective communication between the three brains — the vertical connections are few, and those that do exist are inefficient and slow. MacLean argues that this is the result of our rapid evolutionary spurt about a half-million years back, when our neocortex ballooned with such rapidity that we became top-heavy, victims of a chronic dissociation between upper and lower brains, an imbalance MacLean calls *schizophysiology*. He writes:

> ... one might infer that [the limbic brain] could hardly deal with information in more than a crude way, and was possibly too primitive a brain to analyze language. Yet it might have the capacity to participate in a non-verbal type of symbolism. This would have significant implications as far as symbolism affects the emotional life of the individual. One might imagine, for example, that though the visceral brain could never aspire to conceive of the colour red in terms of a three-letter word or as a specific wave-length of light, it could associate the colour symbolically with such diverse things as blood, fainting, fighting, flowers, etc. — correlations leading to phobias, obsessive-compulsive behavior, etc. Lacking the help and control of the neocortex, its impressions would be discharged without modification into the hypothalamus and lower centres of affective behavior. Considered in the light of Freudian psychology, the old brain would have many of the attributes of the unconscious id. One might argue, however, *that the visceral brain is not at all unconscious (possibly not even in certain stages of sleep), but rather eludes the grasp of the intellect because its animalistic and primitive structure makes it impossible to communicate in verbal terms.* Perhaps it were more proper to say, therefore, it was an animalistic and illiterate brain."

Humans have long been aware of their schizophysiology, which they've characterized in many ways: as a division between higher and lower functions, between conscious and unconscious, between savage and civilized, and so on. One of the most striking symbolic representations is that of Socrates, who in Plato's *Phaedrus* compares the mind to a chariot hitched to two powerful horses. The nearly wild horses seem to be pulling in different directions, and the chariot driver is hard-pressed to keep them under control. One point Socrates' metaphor makes clear is that when the horses and charioteer are working together harmoniously, the speed, power, and range of the horse/chariot/charioteer combination is far greater than for any of the parts: there is a synergistic relationship.

Similarly, there is evidence that despite the well-known difficulties of integrating the levels of the triune brain, it *is* possible to bring the dissociated parts together, with a subsequent enormous increase in capacity, strength, power, and range. This kind of synergistic coordination happens all the time, and is known variously as enlightenment, wholeness, and body/mind unity. It can be seen most frequently in athletes—when all parts of their game come together and their play is at once effortless and astonishing, and they are said to be playing "over their heads"—but all of us have felt it from time to time. For many, these exhilarating moments of vitality and optimism, known by psychologist Abraham Maslow as "peak experiences," are unforgettable reminders of what life is "really" like.

Most importantly for us, there is a large body of evidence that specific techniques exist for bringing about or increasing this vertical unity of the brain. These techniques, including various meditative systems, deep relaxation, biofeedback, trance states, and other approaches, offer, in the words of Dr. Kenneth Pelletier, professor of psychiatry at Langley Porter Neuropsychiatric Institute in San Francisco, "the potential for an individual to clarify the relationships between his physiological and psychological states with unprecedented accuracy and thereby to reduce intra-organismic, psychosomatic stress and the accompanying disorders." With these techniques, he points out, an individual can "establish a clear communication between his higher-order cortical processes and subcortical physical processes in order to induce a more harmonious integration of these functions."[186]

Through this increased communication between neocortex and the older brains, it's possible for us to bring our brains into a state of wholeness or vertical unity—like horses, chariot, and charioteer working together, efficiently and harmoniously—with unprecedented creative power and wisdom, so that Maslow's "peak experiences" come more frequently, more easily, more lastingly. In fact, says writer Colin Wilson, "Once we understand the basic techniques, we can achieve the peak experience as predictably as a good athlete can achieve the high jump."

Well, this is exciting stuff, but is it practical? The unfortunate fact is that while many techniques seem to increase this vertical unity, most of them require more or less lengthy periods of instruction and disciplined daily practice. There is an exception to this, however: the float tank. As a number of recent studies demonstrate, the float tank experience seems to operate directly, rapidly, and dramatically to bring about increased communication and harmony between the vertical levels of the brain, and it does so without prerequisite training, instruction, practice, or arduous self-discipline.

How does floating achieve this? Like the balance it brings to the two hemispheres—synchronous brain waves measurable on the EEG—when you float, certain measurable physiological events occur in the brain that demonstrate increasingly effective communication between the vertical layers. These effects will be discussed at greater length in appropriate chapters of this book, but to summarize a few of the indicators:

≈ Because of the sensory deprivation aspects of being in the tank, the reticular activating system decides our level of stimulation is too low, and turns up the volume on all our senses. As a result we become exquisitely aware of what's going on inside us—thoughts, emotions, physical sensations. By becoming so intensely aware of our internal processes, including autonomic functions like respiration, heartbeat, dilation of blood vessels, and so on, we are able to bring those involuntary functions under conscious control, thereby achieving a unity of reptile brain (RAS), limbic brain (autonomic system), and neocortex (conscious awareness and voluntary control).

≈ Paradoxically, the RAS also seems to treat the experience of floating as a sort of sensory overload on some levels, and responds by turning down the volume on certain functions, causing us to become deeply relaxed, physically immobilized, mentally still, all distractions gone, ordinary thoughts silenced. The result is a distinct, perhaps unique state of being, at once extraordinarily quiet and intensely conscious.

≈ The limbic system responds to floatation by inhibiting the release of hormones and neurotransmitters that have a harmful or stressful effect, such as epinephrine (adrenaline) and norepinephrine, ACTH, and cortisol. At the same time, floating apparently causes the limbic system to *increase* secretion of very beneficial neurochemicals such as the endorphins. Through the release or inhibition of neurochemicals, the limbic system exerts a strong influence over the other parts of the brain, causing us to feel certain emotions (euphoria, reduction in anxiety), and predisposing the neocortex to "think" in certain ways (to become synchronized, to generate theta waves, to increase visualization, to have access to deep memories, and so on).

≈ Conversely, by freeing it from external stimuli, floating allows the neocortex to become more aware of the operation of the limbic system and to assume conscious control over that system; by becoming aware of the effects of certain neurochemicals released by the limbic system, the neocortex can consciously learn to increase or decrease the secretion of those chemicals, much as someone hooked up to a biofeedback machine can learn to raise or lower his own blood pressure. In this we again see the unified and harmonious working of all three levels of the brain: the RAS, which focuses our awareness internally and with single-pointed intensity; the limbic brain, which controls the secretion of neurochemicals that operate the autonomic system; and the neocortex, which (like a charioteer) provides the will and the guidance.

By now the point of the story of Billy the painter and his heroic leap over the banister to coldcock the junkie should be clear. Billy is not the sort of person who would ordinarily get into fights or act impulsively, but in this case he had just emerged from the tank, and all three parts of his brain were operating together. "I don't know what got into me," says Billy, puzzled but exhilarated by his actions. What got into him, of course, was his crocodile and his horse; like an athlete making a perfect play, Billy simply *acted*, all parts of his mind and body directed toward a single goal, and he found himself catapulted into a peak experience of unified self and action.

Our conclusion from Billy's tale is not that floating makes us violent, but that it frees us from the inhibitions the neocortex usually places on our actions, eliminates the ordinary chronic conflict between emotion and reason, intention and action. By uniting the entire brain into a powerful unit, like charioteer and horses, floating enables us to act with a freedom, singleness of purpose, and sense of wholeness we have rarely experienced.

EIGHT

THE BIOCHEMICAL
EXPLANATION

The discovery of the enormous influence that chemical substances in the brain have on our behavior, and the simultaneous discovery that humans can easily and consciously regulate the levels of these neurochemicals in their own brains, have been two of the most exciting, even earthshaking scientific discoveries of the last decade. The brain is no longer what it seemed to be. Dr. David Baltimore, winner of the Nobel Prize for Medicine and Physiology, writes of a friend of his who had devoted many years to intense study of the brain, but then one day decided to give it all up. Baltimore asked why, and the scientist replied that he'd made a wrong bet. He had bet that the brain was a computer and had now seen that the brain is, in truth, an endocrine organ.[9]

An endocrine organ is one that releases internal secretions, and the message of science over the last few years has been that the chemicals secreted by the brain—known as hormones and neurotransmitters—have a profound effect on behavior. Scientists have discovered chemicals associated with sleep, anxiety, aggressiveness, concentration, learning, and so on, right down to fear of the dark.

One revolutionary result of recent findings is that the once-sharp distinction between *hormones* (substances produced by various organs and carried in the bloodstream to other parts of the body where they exert their action for an extended period) and *neurotransmitters* (which as their name implies are chemicals that carry messages between nerve cells, the messages being various moods, emotions, and "states of mind") has become so blurred that it has almost completely broken down. This realization that states of mind (neurotransmitters) and long-lasting chemical actions that control slow processes such as growth and reproduction (hormones) are almost one and the same, says David Baltimore, "gives us some knowledge of the mind/body problem. It says quite clearly that processes within the brain that trigger a hormone release can cause enormous effects on the body." It says, that is, that what we *think* can change our bodies, that there is a quantifiable chemical link between mind and matter, spirit and body, imagination and reality. Spiritual leaders, great thinkers, artists have been saying this very thing for ages, but the fact that hardheaded, hard-research oriented neuroscientists are not just saying it but actually identifying and measuring the very neurochemicals that link idea with matter adds a new legitimacy and urgency to the idea.

For example, biochemists have discovered that certain brain chemicals will tend to make us to feel shy, competitive, afraid, anxious, happy, sleepy, depressed, irritated, and so on. Brain chemicals play a major role in schizophrenia, heart attacks, sleep, stress, and adaptation to stress. Neurochemicals cause us to be sexually aroused, determine the strength of our all-important immune system, cause us to have youthful vitality or feel old and sluggish, help our bodies repair themselves, determine whether we fall in love. By altering or regulating the amounts of these brain chemicals, we can alter and regulate all those behaviors, processes, and mental states.

The remarkable effects of these brain chemicals, and the ways in which floating can help dramatically alter the levels of these chemicals in the brain and body, will be discussed in appropriate chapters of this book. For now, however, the important points are:

Direct Biochemical Benefits.   Tests on the effects of floatation on neurochemicals demonstrate both that floating does have a significant effect on the release of these natural substances, and that the effects have been uniformly beneficial. For example, tests by neuroendocrinologist John Turner and his colleague, psychologist Thomas Fine, of Medical College of Ohio, show that floatation lowers the levels of norepinephrine, epinephrine (also known as adrenaline), cortisol, and ACTH, among others. Elevated levels of these chemicals are directly linked to high levels of stress and stress-related illnesses. Since these neurochemicals have an extraordinary range of effects, let me use cortisol as an example. Among other things, high levels of cortisol have been conclusively linked with "Type A personalities," i.e., people who are aggressive, impatient, and susceptible to heart disease and heart attacks. (Such people produce forty times as much cortisol as Type B personalities—those who are relaxed and virtually immune to heart attacks.) High levels of cortisol have been linked to a number of ailments; they depress the body's immune system, increase the effects of adrenaline on body tissues, and cause fat to be released into the blood and subsequently deposited in the heart (thus contributing to heart disease). A component of the body's fight-or-flight response, the release of cortisol is a reaction to stress, and high levels of the chemical can lead to many stress-related ailments, including depression.

Increased Biochemical Self-regulation. Scientists are now discovering that there is an intimate relationship between consciousness and brain chemistry. To an extent that most scientists would have found unbelievable only a few years ago, we now know that *your attitudes and thoughts change, and can determine, your brain chemistry and your brain chemistry determines what happens in your body.* This revolution is, in essence, a breaking down of the age-old distinction between mind and body, spirit and matter. If wrong mental states beget wrong chemicals beget wrong behavior and disease, the equation can be restated: Right mental states beget beneficial chemicals beget high-level health and well-being.

Candace Pert, a neurochemist at the Biological Psychiatry Branch of the National Institutes of Mental Health, had a part in shaking the scientific world when in 1973 she helped discover the opiate receptor in the brain. Her current work includes creating synthetic drugs and determining their effect on the brain. "In the last twenty years," she says in an interview with science writer Judith Hooper, "psychiatry has come out of the Dark Ages. We know that many forms of mental illness are associated with an imbalance in brain chemicals, and we have drugs that are closely related to those chemicals to treat that imbalance." Such views might seem to tend toward reductionism, the view that the mind is "nothing but" mechanical and chemical interactions. But on the contrary, what she calls her "tinkering around" in the brain's "juices" has convinced her that "consciousness is before the brain."

"It's all in the mind anyway," she says. "Perhaps what this is telling us is that drugs can never be as subtle as our own neurochemicals, which can be released in one spot and not another. Drugs assault the whole brain at once. Who knows, the future psychiatric treatment may consist of auto-hypnosis, meditation, exercise, diet modification, and so on."[101]

The extraordinary thing to take note of here is that the most knowledgeable neuroscientists today are excitedly emphasizing the power of pure consciousness to change the chemistry of the brain. Dr. Pert mentions meditation and auto-hypnosis specifically, but numerous recent studies have clearly shown that floating is far more powerful in influencing brain chemistry than either of these. All current evidence indicates that through effective use of the tank, floaters will be able to alter and influence the chemical secretions of the brain, and thereby affect every aspect of their behavior, including moods, emotions, immune response, and more.

To state this more clearly: We can, through a proper program of floatation, learn how to inhibit the release of certain harmful or unwanted bio-chemicals and stimulate the release of other highly desirable biochemicals. Just as body builders increase the size of their muscles through systematic use of those muscles, so we can develop our ability to release certain chemicals at will, in a process that one scientist calls molecular self-improvement.[4]

Some might find this the stuff of science fiction, but it is well known among neuroscientists that some people are more neurochemically "developed" than others: Each person has an individual body chemistry, with differing amounts of neurotransmitters and hormones available, and larger or smaller numbers of the receptor sites where these neurotransmitters "fit" and are thus able to communicate their messages. Studies show, for example, that heroin addicts have low levels of the body's natural opiates, known as endorphins, in their bodies, and fewer receptor sites where the endorphins can have their pleasure-causing/pain-relieving effects. As the addict continues to take opiates, the number of receptor sites continues to shrink; he or she has to take more and more of "the drug" simply to achieve the same effect, running like crazy to stay in the same place. Thus, one reason for the addictive nature of the opiates (as well as of alcohol) is that they cause the addict's pleasure pathways to deteriorate or wither away. All indications are that some people are born with lower levels of endorphins, or a lower than normal number of endorphin receptors—so their subsequent addictive behavior, whether it involves overeating, smoking, drinking, drugs, sex, or other compulsions, can be seen as a desperate and instinctive attempt to compensate for a certain emptiness, or lack of pleasure, that derives from endorphin deficiencies.

Other people, however, have high levels of endorphins, and/or numerous receptor sites. "All other things being equal," writes Yale biochemist Philip Applewhite, "the differences among people in how happy they are may well reflect differences in how the pleasure center of the hypothalamus functions." Or on differences in the amount of endorphins secreted in certain brain centers: "Those with more endorphins released with certain activities may be happier about any given situation or event in their lives than those with fewer endorphins," according to Applewhite. "That is, doing the same thing may be more pleasurable to one person than another because for that person, more endorphin molecules are released in the brain. Happiness, then, lies not outside the body, but within. Happiness is not an illusion; it is real and has a molecular basis."[4]

People with a greater ability to secrete endorphins experience more pleasure from the same stimulus—be it sex, food, or a beautiful vista—than do those whose pleasure centers and pleasure pathways are less developed. And one way to develop these pleasure centers and to increase the amount and effectiveness of the pleasure-creating neurochemicals is through frequent conscious use. We might say you can "pump endorphins" as a weight lifter pumps iron, with parallel effect.

In addition to demonstrating the chemical basis of addictive behavior, much recent research is revealing that there are neurochemical bases to depression, anxiety, and our ability to fight off disease. Discoveries of direct links between state of mind and the body's immune response have spawned an entire new field known as *psychoneuroimmunology* currently one of the hottest areas of medical research. Float tank researcher Thomas Fine recently told me he believes the most exciting possible use for floating is in developing the strength of the immune system: "One area I'm most interested in is using the tank and mental imagery as a link to *pumping up* the immune system. We need to look at direct links between mental processes, or at least subjective experience, and changes in the immune system." Could a person use the tank to increase directly the power of his or her immune system through increased control of hormonal secretions? "It's highly possible," says Fine.

Weight lifters don't grow such monumental muscles naturally, nor through random heavings of heavy weights; they use a sophisticated program of regular efforts, exercising again and again the muscles they wish to build. Similarly, it is now clear, the way to mold our body chemistry, stimulating or pumping up our positive chemicals and inhibiting the unwanted ones, is through a consciously applied program of self-regulation. It's now apparent that the floatation tank is an ideal environment and tool—at this time *the* ideal environment and tool—to employ for such a program.

NINE

THE BIOFEEDBACK
EXPLANATION

It has always been one of the main assumptions of Western medicine and scientists who deal with the human body that it is necessary to make a distinction between the parts of the body over which we can exercise conscious control—known as the "voluntary" components—and those parts over which we have no conscious control—known as the "involuntary" components.

Among the components of our body thought to be involuntary were: the rhythm and amplitude of our brain waves, healing, blood vessel expansion and contraction, blood pressure, the rate and force of heart contractions, respiratory rate, smooth-muscle tension, the secretion of hormones, the sympathetic nervous system (which acts in the fight-or-flight response, revving us up to deal with a perceived threat), and the parasympathetic nervous system (which has the opposite effect, bringing about the "relaxation response," calming us). In other words, every cell in the body is to a greater or lesser degree subject to "involuntary" control. Like slaves at the mercy of a powerful and unpredictable master who might at one moment use the whip and at the next soothe, we are forever chained to the "involuntary" system. It's no wonder, given this view of the body, that the Western world emphasized the distinction between mind and body: The mind, subject to rational control, was cultivated and valued, while the body, with its unpredictable and involuntary urges, starts, alarms, and breakdowns, was dark, unknown, fearsome, to be resisted and overcome when possible.

Then, in the 1960s, with the development of sophisticated instruments to measure minute changes in the physical functions of laboratory animals, some scientists wondered what would happen to humans who were hooked up to these measuring devices, so that they could observe the activity of their own bodies. The early experiments consisted of measuring subjects' brain waves, and the scientists discovered that within a few minutes most subjects could exercise control over their supposedly involuntary brain waves and could generate large quantities of alpha waves. As research progressed they found that they could "feed back" a signal monitoring not only brain waves but also galvanic skin response (which measures level of arousal), muscular tension, heart rhythms, the activity of internal organs, the temperature of various specific areas of skin—virtually any physical process that could be measured. More tantalizing, they discovered that whatever physical process could be measured, and fed back, could be brought under control. At first cautious, they became increasingly excited by the momentous nature of their discovery. Apparently the ancient distinction between voluntary and involuntary components of the human system had no true basis in fact; somehow humans can exercise control over virtually every cell in their bodies!

This last is no exaggeration. One researcher, John Basmajian, demonstrated that the control we have over our bodies is so sophisticated we can learn to manipulate a *single specific neuron*. Basmajian's subjects, hooked up so they could monitor the firing of their single motor unit neurons, were quickly able to fire off these cells in rhythmic drum rolls, the paradiddles and flourishes played on a single cell out of the hundreds of millions of cells that compose the human body. How could this be done? To locate and control a single cell in the entire body should be more difficult than finding a single grain of sand in a desert.

But while biofeedback demonstrated the remarkable control we have over all parts of our bodies, the practical applications and use of biofeedback have been limited in several ways. For many people, simply being connected to a machine brings about certain physical changes: raised blood pressure, perhaps, inability to concentrate, or increased muscular tension. Heisenberg's uncertainty principle states that in the very act of measurement or observation, enough energy is released to change the system that is being observed. By extension, the principle implies that the act of hooking people up to machines that monitor or observe them will change the people being monitored.

The inherent stress of being attached to machines combines with another stress that is a type of "performance anxiety," similar to that felt by students taking an exam. Because they know they are expected to succeed at something—let's say increasing alpha waves—people with this kind of anxiety "choke," and find it difficult if not impossible to succeed in creating the alpha state. When told that the secret is to let go, many people will *try* to let go until their neck veins bulge and they tremble with tension.

For these and other reasons, biofeedback researchers try to take the subjects off the machines as soon as possible, once they have learned what the correct response "feels" like. The researchers believe it is important for people to learn that *they* are themselves in control, not the machines, and that they can exercise self-regulation even better without the distraction of the machines. Ultimately, the machines are like training wheels, which must be discarded once the subject learns how to ride

It is essential to remember that the way biofeedback machines work is by a process of concentration: By focusing on a single, subtle change in the body, which is being amplified by the machine, we are able to shut off our awareness of the external environment; by turning our attention to an internal signal or state, we tune out the outside world, But this shutting off of external stimuli is exactly what the floatation tank does best. All floaters know the feeling of closing the door of the tank, sinking into the black void, and suddenly being able to hear every heartbeat pounding like a pile driver, blood pulsing through veins that cover the body like an exquisite lacework—every physical sensation is magnified, and because there is no possibility of outside distraction, we are able to focus at will upon any part or system of the body.

Clearly the floatation tank is, as numerous floaters have discovered, a natural biofeedback machine,

To use again the daylight/starlight metaphor, when we enter the tank we "turn off" the sunlight of external awareness, allowing those faint pinpoints of light to emerge as a network of bright stars. The faint body signals that we would ordinarily ignore, or which are drowned out, become powerful presences when we are in the floatation tank. And once those signals are known, it becomes as easy to control and manipulate them as it would be for someone trained on a biofeedback machine, without the drawbacks of biofeedback training.

In fact, evidence now indicates that conscious control over physical processes is gained more easily in floatation because intense awareness of internal signals is combined with the extraordinarily deep state of relaxation provided by the tank. Researchers have consistently noted that the most important prerequisite for attaining control over any body function through biofeedback is relaxation. Much of the early training for people learning to use biofeedback is given over to instruction and practice in deep relaxation. However, this state is not easy to attain in a laboratory setting, wired up to an BEG, EMG (electromyograph), or GSR (galvanic skin response) meter. In the tank, deep relaxation and its accompanying intensified awareness of internal states come rapidly, easily, and reliably. All that remains is for the floater to become aware of whatever internal state he wishes to control—blood pressure, release of endorphins, or muscular tension, for example—to monitor it through the intensified float awareness, and to assume control.

TEN

THE "BENEFITS OF BOREDOM" EXPLANATION

To say that the floatation tank works because it so completely blanks out what we ordinarily think of as external reality may seem like straining after the obvious. But it's important to remember that many of floatation's most powerful effects are achieved less through what *happens* while we are floating than through what doesn't happen: noise, light, normal gravity, other people, a sense of time, and so on.

Though floaters look on the physical and mental effects of sensory restriction as positive, most scientists—not to mention large numbers of people in the mainstream of society—see such isolation as boring if not dangerous. Dr. Lilly writes: "Most people have been programmed to avoid solitude, isolation, and confinement. Television sets in homes are anti-isolation and anti-solitude devices.... Thus, there is a negative attitude toward solitude, isolation, and confinement in most persons."

Some of the negative attitudes have already been mentioned in Chapter Two. A few readers may also recall a widely reprinted article by Woodburn Heron, "The Pathology of Boredom," which first appeared in 1957 in *Scientific American*, "A changing sensory environment seems essential for human beings," Heron wrote. "Without it, the brain ceases to function in an adequate way."[99] (*Pathology*, of course, means the science of diseases, their nature and causes, so even in his title Heron links boredom with disease.) Millions more will remember the episode of *Hawaii Five-O* in which sinister Red Chinese Wo Fat turned trained intelligence agents into quivering jelly by plopping them into isolation tanks: "No man," sneered Wo Fat, "can survive six hours without breaking."

Aside from Lilly, whose explorations of inner space took him on such odd journeys that academic scientists wrote him off as lost, one of the first scientists to challenge these conclusions, and to do so with rigorous work in the laboratory, was Peter Suedfeld, of the University of British Columbia. His influential reconsideration of the "pathology" of sensory isolation was published under the title "The Benefits of Boredom" in the *American Scientist* in 1975. After examining the results of previous experiments in the field, Suedfeld concluded that the reported negative reactions and emotional stress were largely the result of "anxiety-arousing instructions," and were "due more to these frightening peripheral features than to sensory deprivation itself." Suedfeld also pointed out that tests of subjects in sensory deprivation experiments showed significant *beneficial* results from periods of sensory restriction, including "increased visual acuity," "improvements in tactile perception," improvement in auditory sensitivity, increased sensitivity to certain tastes (sweet and bitter). Some improvements in sensory abilities in tests lasted as long as two weeks.

Suedfeld also noted that "significant aspects of perceptual functioning seem to be enhanced by sensory deprivation." Among the beneficial effects he noted were improvements in learning, recall, I.Q. scores, perceptual-motor tasks, enhanced visual concentration, increased short term visual storage, and improved discriminatory learning. All this from an environment Heron claimed would engender a pathological state in the brain and would cause the brain to cease functioning in an "adequate way."

After citing many other cases in which sensory deprivation apparently had beneficial effects, such as helping some of the subjects quit smoking, Suedfeld concluded that sensory isolation influences "in one or another, processes as various as the electrical activity of the brain, biochemical secretions, galvanic skin response, basic sensory and perceptual processes, cognition, motivation, development, group interaction, the relationship between environment and personality characteristics, learning, conformity, attitude change, introspection, and creativity. *This is probably as wide a range of effects as have been investigated in any substantive area by any technique known to psychologists*" (italics mine).[234]

It should be noted that in this article Suedfeld was at times referring to tests done using sensory deprivation chambers, not floatation tanks, yet recent tests indicate that the effects of floatation tanks are as powerful as, or more powerful than, those of the uncomfortable isolation chambers used in these early experiments, Suedfeld himself has in recent years begun working with floatation tanks.

Having remarked that subjects in some of the early sensory deprivation tests seemed open to attitude change, Suedfeld decided to see if these benefits of boredom couldn't he put to productive use in changing harmful behavioral patterns, and settled on cigarette smoking. During his first test utilizing sensory deprivation with smokers, he says he had absolutely no faith that the technique would have any effect on ingrained behavior. However he did a follow-up study after three months, and "lo and behold, we found that those groups in sensory deprivation were smoking almost 40 percent less than the others. This was very encouraging and surprising, Buoyed by this unexpected success, Suedfeld went on to do a whole series of studies of the effects of sensory deprivation on smoking cessation, overcoming phobias, weight reduction, and alcoholism, among others, with extraordinary results. (We will look at Suedfeld's remarkable findings in Chapters Twenty-one, Twenty-two, and Twenty-three.)

In 1983, Suedfeld delivered the keynote address at the First International Conference on REST and Self-Regulation at Denver, and most of the other floatation and sensory deprivation researchers who delivered papers stressed that their work was deeply indebted to Suedfeld's research and ideas. If anyone is an authority on how floating works, it is Suedfeld, so I asked him if he could explain in a general way his understanding of just why it is so successful in changing behavior and attitude. Suedfeld explained what he called the "two factor theory."

Stimulus Hunger.   The first factor to be taken into account, according to Suedfeld, is *stimulus hunger.* Returning to his idea of the benefits of boredom, he pointed out that in a very real way the brain *does* become bored in an environment where there is very little stimulation. And becoming bored, it begins to cast about for something to pay attention to.   Like a habitual reader, deprived of a book, who finds himself desperately reading the back of a cereal box, the person in the isolation chamber or float tank becomes very interested in, and very receptive to, *any* information or stimulation.

Stimulus hunger is an appetite of which the floater is generally, unaware. Far from feeling bored or in desperate need of stimulation, the floater is usually in a state of deep and serene relaxation. Meanwhile, the blissful floater's reticular activating system is deciding that since there is not much sensory stimulation passing through for it to filter and direct to the higher brain, the floater's attention level must he too low. So the RAS turns up the volume or, certain cognitive channels — that is, it heightens arousal and intensifies sensitivity and receptivity to incoming stimuli. But there are no incoming stimuli! So it turns up the volume a bit more ... and so on: stimulus hunger.

Suedfeld, and others who use float tanks to effect behavior and attitude change, do so by allowing enough time to pass for the floater's brain to have developed sufficient stimulus hunger, and then play prerecorded messages to the floater through underwater speakers. When the taped messages arrive in the midst of sensory restriction, the subject's brain pays very close attention and is exceedingly receptive.

Unfreezing Attitudes.   The second factor in the two factor theory has to do with the "frozenness" of attitudes. All habitual, stable attitudes, beliefs, and behavioral patterns are difficult to change, according to Suedfeld, because they are subject to the law of inertia: They tend to continue as they are until some force of greater power is exerted to change them; the attitudes and beliefs are frozen. To change them, you must first unfreeze them. One extremely powerful way to unfreeze attitudes is to enter a float tank.

In part, this is because the floater's deep relaxation makes it seem simply too much of an effort to respond to or offer counterarguments to messages that contradict the frozen attitudes. Another consideration, based on Suedfeld's statistical analysis of changes in belief structures of sensory deprivation subjects, is that subjects undergo a certain amount of cognitive confusion. In the float tank and isolation chamber, says Suedfeld, "well-learned, habitual, stable attitudes and well-learned, habitual, stable behavioral patterns lose their stability and habitualness, so that the system is *unfrozen*, destabilized, becomes confused, and new information then has a much better chance of changing them, because it doesn't have to overcome all that resistance; resistance is weakened."

After attitudes and behavior patterns are unfrozen, new attitudes and behaviors can be substituted for them: "When you're being unfrozen, new information can change the attitude structure into a new pattern by giving you new facts you believe about an issue, or new ideas about how those facts should be evaluated or reacted to. And for new attitudes to become permanent, the new structure has to be *refrozen*. The three stages are unfreezing, changing, and refreezing. This is the theoretical underpinning of the effects of floatation tanks and sensory deprivation on attitude and behavior change." Sensory restriction, says Suedfeld, whether in float tanks or isolation chambers, "is in itself an *unfreezer*."

Deautomatization.   This idea of unfreezing belief structures is paralleled on a neuropsychological level by the concept of *deautomatization*. Psychologists point out that motor behavior tends to become "automatic," and as the physical actions become more automatized, so do the mental acts involved in those actions. An example is the way we come to drive a car automatically, paying virtually no attention to the mental processes or the highly coordinated motor skills involved. Obviously, automatization has great advantages, allowing us to perform an enormous range of mundane tasks without paying attention to them, and enabling us to save our valuable attention for important or novel situations. There are drawbacks, however. Many people have had the experience of getting up, going to work, coming home again, eating dinner, watching TV, getting ready for bed, and at some point coming fully awake and realizing they have gone through the entire day like a robot, on automatic pilot, with no real awareness of their actions or thoughts.

This is not a pleasant realization, and the obvious answer is to break away from automatic actions. Just as belief structures must first be unfrozen, so must automatic actions be deautomatized, a process psychologist Arthur Deikman defines as "the undoing of automatization, presumably by *reinvesting actions and percepts with attention*," and "an undoing of the usual ways of perceiving and thinking due to the special way that attention is being used." [56] When people are able to deautomatize themselves, Deikman points out, they are filled with a powerful feeling of intensified sensory perceptions. William Blake spoke of "cleansing the doors of perception," and Deikman cites other mystics who have experienced a "new vision," a clarification of everything seen.

How is this deautomatization achieved? Deikman examines several techniques, including contemplative meditation, but focuses on the idea of "renunciation," including "isolation and silence." *Isolation and silence* sounds something like the float tank, but Deikman continues: "To the extent that perceptual and cognitive structures require the 'nutriment' of their accustomed stimuli for adequate functioning, renunciation would be expected to weaken and even disrupt these structures, thus tending to produce an unusual experience. Such an isolation from nutritive stimuli probably occurs internally as well." This, of course, is reminiscent of unfreezing and of stimulus hunger. It may be, says Deikman, that meditation "creates temporary stimulus barriers producing a functional state of sensory isolation. On the basis of sensory isolation experiments it would be expected that long-term deprivation ... of a particular class of stimulus 'nutriment' would cause an alteration in those functions previously established to deal with that class of stimuli. These alterations seem to be a type of deautomatization.... Thus, *renunciation alone can be viewed as producing deautomatization*" (italics mine). That is, the isolation tank experience ("renunciation") produces deautomatization. On a sensory level, this explains why the world seems so fresh, colors so bright, our senses so keen, when we emerge from the tank. Our habitual or automatic ways of perceiving the world have been disrupted; we perceive things with a new intensity of attention. The world has become new.

ELEVEN

THE RELAXATION
RESPONSE EXPLANATION

We all know what stress is. Though we might not be able to explain the physiological process, we're quite clear about our feelings. We talk about sweaty
palms, chills down the spine, quivering like a leaf, getting cold feet, being
tight-assed, having butterflies in the stomach, or receiving a shot of adrenaline. Many use these phrases with the belief that they're just figures of speech,
apt clichés, not realizing that they are describing with poetic exactness very
real physiological processes, all of which are part of an unconscious, reflexive
reaction to stress known as the fight-or-flight response.

This reaction is initiated and carried out by the so-called involuntary nervous system. This system, also known as the autonomic nervous system, has
two distinct but interdependent parts, each of which operates to mobilize the
body's resources in quite different ways, one by spending, one by saving: the
first, by pouring out the body's energy in actions; the second, by conserving
and storing energy. The first, the *sympathetic nervous system*, is activated during the fight-or-flight response, in several distinct steps. Something happens
in the external world; it is conveyed to the hypothalamus, which interprets it
as a threat requiring response, and releases several neurochemicals. Some of
these chemicals go to the nearby pituitary, where they trigger the release of
the hormone ACTH (adrenocorticotropic hormone), which is rapidly carried
through the bloodstream to the adrenal glands, where it triggers the release
of cortisol. Cortisol causes an increase in blood sugar and accelerates the
body's metabolism in various ways. Meanwhile, other chemicals from the
hypothalamus go directly to the adrenals, triggering an outpouring of epinephrine (adrenaline) and norepinephrine, thus releasing more blood sugar
and increasing the heart rate, respiration, and blood pressure. These chemical chain reactions and physiological changes are all directed toward one goal:
preparing the body with great speed to deal with some external threat. In
rapid order, blood pressure rises; blood flow is shifted away from the diges-
tive system and the periphery of the body to the heart and trunk muscles; res-

piration becomes shallow and rapid; the pelvis becomes rigid, anus tight, genitals numb; palms sweat; muscles become so tense we often tremble; oxygen consumption increases; body temperature rises; and as stress hormones flood through the system we respond with an "adrenaline rush," that jolt of surging energy that enables a tiny woman to lift an automobile off her trapped husband. We are in what Dr. Kenneth Pelletier calls "an intense, overall state of undifferentiated hyperarousal."[186]

In rats, rabbits, apes, or humans, the fight-or-flight response is a marvelously efficient evolutionary mechanism for enabling an animal to deal with a threat to its security. The complex biochemical and neurophysical actions enable the body to mobilize quickly its strengths and powers for defense, aggression, or flight. In situations of real threat, the animal can respond with fight or flight and, having discharged the energy of the automatic response, can (if it has survived) dive into its safe home or burrow and let the aftereffects of the response fade away. After we have delivered a speech, or narrowly avoided a car accident, or emerged from a barroom punch-out, we need time to recover, to sit back, still trembling, heart still pounding, breathing shallow, and let the emergency juices flow out of us. And as they do, we feel our muscles relax, breathing deepen, entire body seem to soften with a feeling of delicious release and relief, as we realize that the threat is over, and even more, *the threat is over and I'm still alive!*

But times have changed, and we civilized folk rarely confront threatening situations that can be dealt with so clearly. Our daily threats are more likely to consist of sitting next to some loud-talking idiot in a restaurant and wishing we could strangle the motormouth as we try to maintain a calm exterior in an important business negotiation.

Most stress-inducing stimuli we confront today are subtle, unidentifiable, or indirect: noise and air pollution; business, social, and family pressures; ambiguous civilized conflicts; environmental carcinogens; potential nuclear war; unemployment; constant fears of street crime; general antagonism between the sexes; and other abstract and insidious stressors. "Habitual, chronic, unabated stress has replaced such immediate threats as loss of life, starvation, or territorial combat which characterized the stresses of primitive man and animals," says Pelletier, concluding that contemporary man is in "a perpetual state of nonspecific arousal."[186]

The results of such unrelieved stress have been noted by endocrinologist Hans Selye, who described the specific series of processes by which we react to stress, a progression he called the General Adaptation Syndrome (G.A.S.).[214] This syndrome, according to Selye, consists of three stages: alarm, resistance, and exhaustion. The alarm is our initial reaction to a stressor, the dramatic fight-or-flight mobilization of the body's entire stress mechanism. In resistance, our bodies focus their attention on the specific point at which stress is attacking us, and the resistance shifts to those organs that are best capable of handling the threat. However, because our resources are diverted toward dealing with the specific stress, our general resistance to disease is weakened. If the threat is prolonged, our resources become exhausted, the immune system becomes depleted, and the body begins to break down, especially the organ or system that is handling the stressor.

Ultimately, when prolonged stress is not overcome, the body develops symptoms such as the shrinking of the thymus, spleen, and the lymph nodes; the disappearance of certain white blood cells; and stomach or duodenal ulcers. Just as an overworked machine breaks down at its weakest point, the human body appears to break down at its weakest spot, the "target organ," which varies from person to person depending on heredity and life history.

Burn-out. To resist this stress, each person apparently has a certain amount of hereditary "adaptation energy." Some people start out with a lot, others with less. Once this allotted amount of adaptation energy has been expended in resisting stress, however, it is gone for good, according to Selye: Like a nation's oil deposits, it can be used only once and can't be replenished. So people who have stumbled into a stressful marriage, say, or been subject to prolonged torture will use up their adaptation energy rapidly, will age quickly, and be more liable to disease. Many such people are correctly described as being burned out.

To add to the problem, man is unlike the other animals in that he has developed an enlarged cortex, which has to some degree taken over control of the other parts of the brain. So while our reptile brain and limbic system are reacting to stress with a powerful fight-or-flight response, our new cortex is often imposing a kind of censorship on our actions. This censorship is based on moral precepts that have no biological basis at all but are purely creations of our own minds. Thus, rather than recognizing stress symptoms for what they are, we often try to desensitize ourselves to or dissociate ourselves from the symptoms. When people are so frightened that they can't eat, they tell themselves they have indigestion; when anxiety robs them of sleep, they talk about insomnia; the chronic tight back that is a reaction to deep terror is referred to as a back problem.

Ironically, these reactions, which are actually only normal responses to stress, are perceived by the sufferers as symptoms of disease which increases their anxiety, which in turn increases the symptoms, in a self-feeding cycle of ever more serious symptoms and reactions. While our normal reaction to stress is to run or to violently defend ourselves, our society is based on restraining these impulses to action. However, as Pelletier points out, "Immobility is interpreted by the subcortex as evidence of insufficient preparation for fight or flight and it initiates more vigorous biochemical reactions. Subjectively the individual experiences this biochemical alteration as mounting tension. The termination or interruption of this highly destructive cycle may be the key to alleviating psychosomatic disorders."

But how can we interrupt this progressively degenerative cycle? According to Pelletier, "To restore an individual's capacity to identify, react to, and then relax from stressful conditions appears to be the critical point of resolution. Such an intervention based upon individual autoregulation is both necessary and possible."[186]

Fight or Flight or Float

The idea of alleviating psychosomatic disorders by breaking the vicious cycle of stress and stress reaction brings us right to the floatation tank. While the stress relief of the tank works on a number of levels simultaneously, one obvious fact is that entering the floatation tank removes you from most stressors, both the primary stressor and secondary environmental stresses. In the tank there is no noise, no light, no other people, nothing to do, and nothing that needs to be or can be done. Like that time after the fight or the near accident, when you needed someplace just to sit and wind down, the tank is the perfect recovery-from-stress spot. There, with no possible threat from the outside world, your body slows down, the flood of chemicals that has jangled your nerves is eliminated, and your body chemistry returns to normal. And just as when, after some stressful moment, your heightened arousal gives way to a feeling of deep calmness, so in the tank the deepening relaxation of your body and brain is perceived as a delicious sensation of peace, well-being, exhilaration: *I have survived and I am alive!*

Another important factor: To relax fully, an individual must, as Pelletier says, have the capacity to "identify, react to, and then relax from stressful conditions." Unfortunately, few people can find the time or place in this stressful society for serious contemplation of their lives and identification of the causes of their problems. For some with large amounts of time and money, psychoanalysis has attempted to fulfill this function. But the fact remains that our society places little value on sitting alone, silently, contemplating our lives, examining ourselves for tension, and seeking out its immediate and indirect causes.

The floatation tank, removing all external distractions, provides the floater with an unhurried, unpressured opportunity to examine his or her life from a distance, to get a comparatively objective view of any situation, to interrupt the cycle of fight-or-flight tension before it gets out of control, and before it is too late.

The Relaxation Response

That the floatation tank offers a relatively stress-free environment in which to escape temporarily from stressful external stimuli and free your system from its chronic state of arousal makes it a useful and life enhancing tool. But if that were *all* it did, the floatation tank would be essentially a passive tool, and entering a tank would be little different from sitting quietly in a dark room, While the absence of stress is desirable in itself, it doesn't necessarily bring about the presence of its opposite, relaxation.

The floatation tank goes far beyond the passive. Scientists have now proved that floating activates a physiological response that is parallel to, and as powerful as, the stressful one of fight or flight. This response mobilizes the body's resources to bring about an active, alert, positive, and beneficial state of deep relaxation.

The description of relaxation as a distinct, active, and alert state may strike you as paradoxical or nonsensical. After all, we get "relaxed" when we're spaced out in front of the tube, or catching some rays on the beach, out fishing, or just goofing off, hacking around, laid back—none of which are particularly distinct, active or alert states. One of the unfortunate legacies of the Judeo-Christian heritage that still permeates our culture is the tendency to look on relaxation as something opposed to productive activity. If you're relaxed, then *ipso facto* you're not doing anything worthwhile. So, with its connotations of laziness, lethargy, and wasting time, we look on relaxation as a luxury, something unimportant or even a bit shameful, when in truth our normal life puts us into such a state of chronic tension and arousal that relaxation is absolutely essential to maintaining our mental and physical health.

Another misconception in our accepted view is that relaxation is something that just happens whenever we stop doing "productive" things or get away from overtly stressful situations—all we have to do is stop working and presto! we're relaxed. In reality, as Pelletier points out, "The reacquisition of a harmonious state of mind-body integration requires both effort and training to establish and sustain."[186] It is no more natural to be in a state of true relaxation than it is to be in a state of fight-or-flight arousal. Like fight or flight, relaxation is a distinct physiological response that involves the coordinated activities of a large part of our nervous system.

The fight-or-flight response, initiated by the hypothalamus, involves the activities of the part of the autonomic nervous system that is called the sympathetic nervous system. There is a second part of the autonomic system, also regulated by the hypothalamus: the *parasympathetic nervous system*. Like a mirror image of the sympathetic system, the parasympathetic works by decreasing muscular tension and releasing biochemicals that fill the body with a sense of well-being, pleasure, safety, and euphoria. While the sympathetic system is mainly involved in *spending*, in mobilizing our bodies for outward activity, muscular exertion, and the use of large amounts of energy, the parasympathetic system is mainly involved in *saving*, in the housekeeping work of the body, and focuses on nourishing and repairing our tissues, excreting wastes, relaxing, and building up and storing energy.

The effects of the parasympathetic response are as striking as those of the sympathetic response, though generally opposite, and include a reduction in heart rate, blood pressure, and sweating, increased functioning of the gastrointestinal tract, a change in the predominant type of brain-wave activity from beta waves to alpha and theta waves, the relaxation of muscles, decreased respiratory rate, decreased use of oxygen, decrease of blood lactate. Like our vast repertoire of stock phrases to describe the fight-or-flight state, we have numerous colorful expressions for the parasympathetic response that we often assume to be simply useful metaphors but which are quite exact and apt: People feel "warmth in their veins," are "glowing" and "positively radiant"; some people "soften our hearts." In this state we become "loose," or "solid as a rock," and "breathe easy."

Herbert Benson of Harvard Medical School made a study of this parasympathetic reaction and, counterposing it to the fight-or-flight response, named it The Relaxation Response. Benson and his colleagues found that this response, while produced by the activation of part of our involuntary system, can be quite easily elicited through conscious use of certain specific techniques, which can be learned and used by anyone.

Benson and his colleagues studied ancient meditative disciplines as well as such modern systems as Transcendental Meditation and the recent discoveries in biofeedback, and concluded that they all worked by eliciting the relaxation response, and that they all were able to do so by using certain techniques in combination. By eliminating nonessential elements and finding the common roots of all the techniques, Benson concluded that there are four preconditions for eliciting the relaxation response:

(1) Mental Device—There should be a constant stimulus e.g., a sound, word, or phrase repeated silently or audibly, or fixed gazing at an object. The purpose of these procedures is to shift from logical, externally oriented thought. (2) Passive Attitude—If distracting thoughts do occur during the repetition or gazing, they should be disregarded and one's attention should be redirected to the technique.... (3) Decreased Muscle Tonus.—The subject should be in a comfortable posture so that minimal muscular work is required. (4) Quiet Environment—A quiet environment with decreased environmental stimuli should be chosen.[21]

Benson, and numerous other researchers who have since studied the relaxation response, have found it quite effective in alleviating virtually every stress-related disease and problem (and most experts estimate that 85 to 90 percent of all illness today is stress-related), including high blood pressure, ulcers, asthma, anxiety, fatigue, and heart disease. In addition, anyone who regularly elicits the relaxation response seems to profit with increased emotional, mental, and physical strength and stability; decreased consumption of drugs, cigarettes, and alcohol; and increased ability to cope with the stresses of everyday life.

Something that is so good for you and makes you feel so good—there's got to be a catch, right? Yes. The catch is, as millions of people have found out who have at one time or another tried to meditate, it is not as easy as it sounds. Meditation, or any technique for eliciting the relaxation response, demands discipline: You must learn the technique, and then you must stick to it long enough for it to begin to have an effect. Many people require several weeks of daily practice before they can reach the state of physical quietness that means success. Many, lacking either faith or discipline, or simply under too much stress, give up rather quickly. In many cases they are so irritated by their apparent inability to learn this "simple" technique that their level of stress has been increased. For some who are already nervous, tense, suffering from a stress-related illness, the idea that they should sit quietly and calm their minds long enough to become deeply relaxed seems a bad joke. Research has shown that a large number of people today lead lives of such habitual tension and chronic low-level stress that they have *never in their adult lives* experienced true relaxation. It's not surprising that large numbers of people are unable to reach states of relaxation through self-help techniques: Telling most people to relax is like sending them out in search of a frumious bandersnatch. They're not going to be able to find it unless they know what it is.

Easy Meditation. For these people, and for anyone interested in eliciting the relaxation response, the floatation tank is the perfect tool. A look through the latest research makes it clear: *The floatation tank is the easiest, most rapid, most foolproof and failure-free method of obtaining the beneficial mental and physical effects of the relaxation response yet discovered.*

Scientific evidence—mentioning only studies dealing with physiological effects linked with the parasympathetic response—has shown that a single float as short as forty-five minutes can:

≈ Significantly decrease blood pressure, heart rate, oxygen consumption, blood lactate, and muscular tension
≈ Increase production of alpha and theta waves in the brain, and bring about synchronous and symmetrical rhythms throughout the cortex
≈ Increase circulation to the extremities and the gastrointestinal system
≈ Decrease the levels of such fight-or-flight biochemicals as epinephrine, norepinephrine, ACTH, and cortisol.

Some of the most fascinating work in this context is that of neuro-endocrinologist John Turner and psychologist Thomas Fine of the Medical College of Ohio. They have done extensive testing of the effects of floating on hormones and other neurochemicals. They discovered that a single float activated the relaxation response, and more importantly, that it did so by very specifically *countering* the effects of the fight-or-flight response. That is, they found that floating significantly lowered all the correlates of the adrenal-sympathetic arousal state, such as ACTH, adrenaline, and cortisol; and further, that a series of floats increased the effectiveness of the relaxation response. Most significantly, they found that floating had a strong "maintenance effect"—the lowering of adrenal-sympathetic (fight-or-flight) activity went on for many days after the subject's last float. This led them to conclude, in the words of Turner, that floating "could alter the set points in the endocrine homeostatic mechanism so that the individual would be experiencing a lower adrenal activation state. It would essentially be associated with a greater degree of relaxation."[252] This is striking and significant, since it means that the beneficial effects of floating are not just temporary, but have the effect of altering the metabolism (or homeostatic set-points), essentially damping down the fight-or-flight response, and pumping up the relaxation response.

Since the control center of what Fine and Turner call "the endocrine homeostatic mechanism" is the hypothalamus, another way of stating this is that floating apparently makes the hypothalamus more resistant to stress, and does so for long periods of time. Says Yale biochemist Philip Applewhite, "The hypothalamus brain program that recognizes stress when it comes in over the nerves is certainly a source of variability. Some people may feel stressed when not much has happened to them; they have a low tolerance for stress. For others it may take considerably more stress before the hypothalamus identifies it as such; these people have a high tolerance for stress."[4] According to the research of Fine and Turner, floating "alters the set-point in the endocrine homeostatic mechanism so that the individual would be experiencing a lower adrenal activation state."[252] That is, *floating is a way of increasing our tolerance for stress.*

What's fascinating about these studies, and is borne out in my interviews with floaters, is that this extraordinarily deep relaxation is a product of the tank experience itself, not the result of some conscious effort or technique on the part of the floaters. It just happens. Turner and Fine concluded one of their papers with a comparison of floatation with other relaxation techniques:

> These [other] techniques have the individual elicit relaxation utilizing some internal strategy with or without external feedback as to the success of the strategy. In contrast [floatation tank] relaxation utilizes an environment to induce relaxation with the individual passively experiencing the process... The controlled repeated experiences of this effortless passive relaxation provided by the [tank] may provide an advantage over these other methods requiring a trial and error approach to the deep relaxation state.[74]

This "effortless" aspect of floatation is important, because it means that even those people who have never felt deep relaxation, and therefore don't really know what it is, are enabled to experience the state. It usually happens during the first float, and is unmistakable. Many discover for the first time what it means to release all muscular tension, and they can see how habitually tense they have been; they understand clearly that relaxation is not lethargy or the simple absence of overt stress, but a distinct and beneficial state.

"I never knew!" shouted my friend Courtney as soon as I picked up the phone. An experienced meditator, Courtney is a novelist, intensely involved in finishing his magnum opus, under a lot of stress. I had recommended floating to him, and he'd halfheartedly agreed to try. Now he was excitedly telling me about his first float, "I'd always talked about stress and tension," he said, "but I never knew how powerful it was, how much energy and strength it's sapping all the time. I guess I never knew what it felt like *not* to be tense. There in the tank it all *melted* and I just started laughing because I suddenly realized how much tightness I'd been carrying around with me all my life, and how incredibly pleasant it is to be free of it. When I got out I realized, my God, there's no reason I can't stay like this all the time!"

Judging from current research, it's evident that on virtually every scale used to assess relaxation, floatation tanks work; not only do they bring about a state of uniquely deep relaxation, but they do so with unmatched speed, safety, and certainty. John Stanley, William Francis, and Heidi Berres, of Lawrence University, undertook a study on the effects of floating on cognitive tasks, comparing the cognitive abilities of three separate groups: a float group, a meditation group, and a control group that neither floated nor meditated but simply sat quietly relaxed in a dark room. Among their interesting results (the floaters significantly lowered their blood pressure and decreased their muscle tension as measured on an electromyograph [EMG]), were the analysis of a subjective relaxation test. All subjects were asked to evaluate how relaxed they were, and the responses showed that floaters considered themselves much more relaxed than the meditators did. The study concluded that the effects of floating "go beyond those of meditation or simple relaxation in a quiet room." [228]

What makes the tank such an unparalleled tool for eliciting the relaxation response? One way of answering this question is to refer to Herbert Benson's list of four essential elements. The first precondition is some "constant stimulus." As Robert Ornstein points out in his classic study *On the Psychology of Meditation*, this restriction of attention to a single thing is a characteristic of most meditative practices, such as chanting, repeating a prayer or mantra, staring at a mandala, counting breaths: "It seems that a consequence of the structure of our central nervous system is that if awareness is restricted to one unchanging source of stimulation, a 'turning off' of consciousness of the external world follows." All these "constant stimulus" techniques, Ornstein contends, are ways of "turning off" the external environment, "inducing a central state in the nervous system equivalent to that of no external stimulation." [171]

But rather than inducing a state *equivalent* to no external stimulation, the tank puts the floater directly into the *actual* state of no external stimulation. Seen in this way, the various methods by which meditative techniques laboriously attempt to short-circuit the nervous system into "turning off' external awareness are simply indirect attempts to do what the floatation tank does directly.

Benson's second essential element, a passive attitude, ignoring distractions, is another state more easily and completely attained in the floatation tank. External distractions are eliminated, and with nothing outside itself to hold on to, the active mind quickly tires and gives up.

Benson's third precondition for the relaxation response, decreased muscle tonus, is quickly attained in the tank, where reduction of the stresses of gravity and the absence of hard surfaces to cause discomfort bring about a degree of muscular relaxation that is difficult, if not impossible, to match within Earth's atmosphere.

The fourth essential element, "decreased environmental stimuli," is self-evident: The floatation tank decreases environmental stimuli as much as is feasible outside of complicated and expensive sensory deprivation environments that are only possible in a specially equipped laboratory setting. Other techniques require dedication, discipline, and often much work before the practitioner is able to elicit the relaxation response at will. Whoever steps into a floatation tank will find the relaxation response activated effortlessly, within minutes.

Another key to floating's power in activating the relaxation response is that it largely eliminates the overriding cause of stress. What is this cause? Not simply danger, threat, or the need to flee, since even joyful events are stressful. George Mandler, professor of psychology at the University of California, and director of the Center for Human Information Processing, characterizes the essence of stress as *interruption*, which he describes as "a discrepancy between one's expectations and the actual evidence from the world," and a "deviation from the expected." When such an interruption happens, he says, "whenever an action cannot be brought to completion, whenever a plan is not quite brought to its end," whenever we interact with reality and find that *something is different*, our sympathetic system is aroused, and we experience stress.

"From an evolutionary point of view," says Mandler, "it makes very good sense to construct an organism that reacts significantly and distinctively when the world is not the way it has been in the past. And in that sense the autonomic nervous system doesn't just have an internal function, it also alerts the organism to something important going on; the world is not the way it was." [166]

The problem is that today the world is almost *never* the way it was; life is one long deviation from the expected. What Mandler calls interruption has become almost constant, and the result is constant sympathetic arousal, constant stress. But in the tank, the "actual evidence from the world" is eliminated, so there can be no conflict between it and our expectations. There are no actions to be brought to completion, no plans to be brought to their ends. In an unchanging environment, we do not discover that *something is different;* inside the tank the world is always the way it was. In a state of deep relaxation, in the constant absence of light, sound, gravity, movement, and temperature variations, there are (speaking in ideal terms) no interruptions, no deviations from expectations, no discrepancies between the way things are and the way we intend them to be. There is nothing to cause the sympathetic system to become aroused, and as a result, no stress.

TWELVE

THE VISUALIZATION EXPLANATION

In one of the most famous experiments in psychology, researcher Alan Richardson divided his schoolboy subjects into three groups. The boys of each group were tested on their skills at sinking a basketball from the free-throw line. The first group was then told to practice shooting free throws every day. The second group was told that they should not practice shooting at all, but rather should *visualize* themselves shooting the basketball. The third group was told not to practice or visualize at all.

At the end of twenty days the groups were reassembled and tested. The non-practicing, non-visualizing group predictably showed no improvement. The group which had practiced every day showed a 24 percent improvement. The ones who had practiced only in the mind's eye showed an improvement of 23 percent.[196] These remarkable results—demonstrating that mental practice brought almost as much improvement as actual physical practice—have been confirmed again and again in similar tests in recent years.

Dr. O. Carl Simonton, director of the Cancer Counseling and Research Center in Fort Worth, Texas, tells his patients—most of them diagnosed as terminal cancer cases—to visualize their bodies successfully resisting and conquering the cancer, "If you are receiving radiation treatment," he counsels, "picture it as a beam of millions of bullets of energy hitting any cells in its path." White blood cells can be seen in the mind's eye as "a vast army," or as valiant White Knights, or powerful polar bears tearing apart and devouring the cancer cells. Statistical studies of Simonton's patients show that those who use visualization and relaxation live twice as long after the diagnosis of cancer as those who do not. Many recover completely through that inexplicable phenomenon known as spontaneous remission.

What You See Is What You Get
Manipulation of mental imagery is probably the most ancient technique for mobilizing inner energies for self-healing and self-regulation. I suspect that

the earliest images that have come down to us from our ancient ancestors—
the cave paintings found in southern France and Spain—were used as tools
for guided visualization. We know that the shamans and healers of primitive
cultures are able to see themselves leaving their bodies and going on extraordinary journeys, to reach the source of wisdom and return with its healing
power. But visualization is not inherently spiritual, associated only with mystical practices or primitive mentalities. Aristotle contended that mental
imagery was not merely one element of thought, but the absolutely essential
element: "It is impossible even to think without a mental picture," he wrote.
"The same affection is involved in thinking as in drawing a diagram." Albert
Einstein, when asked what kind of thinking he used to produce his creative
work, replied, "The words or the language, as they are written or spoken, do
not seem to play any role in my mechanism of thought. The psychical enti-
ties which seem to serve as elements in thought are certain signs and more or
less clear images which can be 'voluntarily' reproduced and combined."[30]

Biofeedback researchers have found that the most effective way of manipulating any body process is through visualization: Migraine sufferers who
want to increase the blood flow and warmth of their hands (which generally
alleviates migraines) do so easily when they visualize their hands dipped in
hot water or resting on the hot sand of a beach. People with chronic muscular tensions can visualize their muscles as ropes or tightly twisted towels
becoming untwisted, limp. In fact, C. Maxwell Cade, who has conducted
biofeedback research on more than four thousand subjects, says, flatly, *"The
ability to think in sensory images instead of in words is as absolutely essential first step
toward the mastery of higher states of consciousness, self-control of pain, etc."* [40]

Mental images seem to be the natural mode of thought, and recent studies show that our minds can remember visual images much better than words
or numbers—so much so that it's now thought that our capabilities for visual recognition are practically perfect. In one experiment, subjects were shown
thousands of slides, one every ten seconds, over a period of days. Later the
slides were mixed with others that the subjects hadn't seen, and were shown
to the subjects at a rate as fast as one every second, hour after hour, and at
times were even shown in mirror image or backward, yet the subject recognized virtually every image that had been shown to him before. The experimenter concluded: "These experiments ... suggest that recognition of pictures
is essentially perfect."[227]

This extraordinary capacity for retaining and manipulating mental
images is one of our most powerful gifts. The power that mental images exert
over us is even more remarkable. Exactly how mental images are able to cause

such profound effects on our system is still a mystery, but many students of consciousness have observed that vivid mental images seem to be accepted by our bodies as being real. This is one way of viewing the basketball experiments: By holding strong images of successfully shooting basketballs, the mind was able to convince the body that the mental images were actually happening, and the body "learned" from this mental picture.

Dr. Edmund Jacobson, a physiologist and the developer of Progressive Relaxation therapy, established this link between mental image and body by having people visualize themselves running. He then used a machine to measure their minute muscular contractions, which he found to be of the type the subjects would have produced if they had actually been running.[113,114] For some reason, when the mind perceives something as happening, it tends to generate organic changes.

Just how remarkable some of those organic changes can be is seen in the hundreds of spontaneous remissions brought about by the visualization techniques of O. Carl Simonton. Less crucial, but equally striking, are the numerous meticulously documented cases of breast enlargement in groups of women using visualization. Each study used a different visualization technique: In one, the women were told to visualize a warm towel over their breasts, with a heat lamp shining down on them. Other groups visualized themselves as they would like to be. Still others visualized blood and energy flowing into their breasts. In all the studies the increase in breast size was significant. The average increase in breast measurement was slightly under one and a half inches in one study, two inches in another. One carefully controlled study was limited to twelve weeks, with an average bust increase of 2.1 inches; and at the same time many of the women reported that they had lost weight, so the increase was not the result of extra pounds.[136,169,261,262]

Some may feel ambivalent about the value of investing mental energy in breast enlargement. But the unquestionable implication of these studies is that mental imagery has power to bring about dramatic and rapid organic change. And what is true for breast enlargement is also true for losing weight or overcoming illness. Quite literally, what you "see" is what you get.

Researchers in the field of mental imagery now believe that about 15 percent of all people are "visualizers" who experience virtually constant, vivid mental imagery; another 1.5 percent of the population are "verbalizers," operating mostly (but not entirely) in a world of words and verbal thoughts, ideas, and structures. The remaining 70 percent lie on a spectrum between these two types. Tests made from the earliest days of infancy through adulthood show that males are consistently superior to females in visualization and visual-spatial ability, though both males and females show a similar distribution of verbalizers and visualizers. Studies show that high visualizers breathe more regularly than verbalizers, and that verbalizers breathe more regularly than they normally do when doing spatial tasks that require visualization. Writer Gordon Rattray Taylor cites studies showing that "high imagers are more relaxed, more creative, more mature, and more flexible than low-imagers.... We have a clue in the fact that absence of imagery is correlated with strong defences against impulse."[246]

As for the value of imagery, aside from the life-enhancing qualities of visualization and the relaxed physical state that seems to accompany it, there are definite practical advantages. Many studies have shown clearly that visual imagery is associated with the ability to remember: The stronger your mental imagery, the less effort you will need to take in and commit to memory an idea or event. People with "supermemories" are able to perform their feats through mental images. With words, linked end to end like boxcars, we can understand only in linear fashion, one bit at a time, while with imagery we can assimilate an entire scene, event, or complex relationship. Visualization is also a crucial element of creativity; by "seeing" things which have never been, or visualizing events before they have taken place, we can truly invent the future, just as we can invent a work of art or a new machine. History is studded with stories of creative geniuses who first encountered their reality-changing ideas in the form of visions, or mental images.

Professor Thomas Taylor of Texas A & M recently conducted a fascinating test of the effects of floating on learning and thinking. Taylor had tested subject groups to see which were visualizers and which were verbalizers, and concluded: "When the same learning records are analyzed on the basis of persons who are basically 'visualizers' versus those who are primarily 'conceptualizers' (non-visual thinkers), a greater degree of learning occurred in the visual than in the non-visual group."[248] Taylor also noted that the float group appeared to visualize better than the non-float group, and produced significantly higher amounts of theta waves, which are known to be associated with strong mental imagery.

If you are a poor visualizer or believe that you have no ability to see pictures in your mind, it is important to remember that in reality you are able to produce imagery. "There is a virtual unanimity among imagery researchers," writes psychologist Robert Sommer, "that everyone has the capacity to think visually. This is as innate a potential as drawing or building or the use of language, or any other skill that develops through practice. If the potential is there, there is the possibility of improvement through training. Not all people can become super-imagers, any more than they will be able to sketch like Leonardo ... but everyone has the potential to improve the pungency of his or her thinking over what it presently is."[224] The ability to experience and manipulate clear inner imagery can be increased dramatically through practice and experience. And the best environment that has yet been created for experiencing mental imagery at its most intense and vivid, and for manipulating mental imagery, is the floatation tank.

The floatation tank is the optimal environment for visualization because the relaxation it ensures is so profound that the brain soon begins to generate an unprecedented amount of very slow, strong, rhythmical theta waves, which are associated with vivid, lifelike hypnagogic images. All methods of visualization used throughout history—the yogi's and monk's relaxed motionless lotus posture, the shaman's drug-induced catatonia—have emphasized that a state of deep relaxation is essential to successful visualization. In the tank, deep relaxation and strong mental imagery come spontaneously and effortlessly.

Floaters are often amused by people who ask them, "But isn't it boring? I mean, just floating around in a dark box, with *nothing happening?*" Far from being boring, for just about everyone who gets into the tank, floating is great fun. The question arises: *Why?* Which leads to another, deeper question: Just what exactly constitutes fun? What are the elements of enjoyment?

These are important questions, especially for floaters, since so much of what they value about floating revolves around having fun doing something many people look on with some trepidation, or at least with ambiguous feelings. The second question intrigued Mihaly Csikszentmihalyi, a professor in the Department of Behavioral Science at the University of Chicago. What, he wondered, is *intrinsically rewarding?* That is, behavior that is engaged in not for external rewards, "not as compensation for past desires, not as preparation for future needs, but as an ongoing process which provides rewarding experiences in the present."

To study this *autotelic* behavior (from the Greek *auto:* self, and *telos:* goal), Csikszentmihalyi interviewed and studied chess players, composers, dancers, basketball players, rock climbers, surgeons, and others who did things they deeply enjoyed. His first conclusion, as he explains it in his book *Beyond Boredom and Anxiety,* was that "The underlying similarity that cuts across these autotelic activities ... is that they all give participants a sense of discovery, exploration, problem solution—in other words, a feeling of novelty and challenge." The outcome of an autotelic activity is uncertain ("Like exploring a strange place") but the actor is potentially capable of controlling it.

After noticing that his informants frequently described their experiences of enjoyment by using the same word, "flow," Dr. Csikszentmihalyi abandoned the term autotelic experience:

> From here on, we shall refer to this peculiar dynamic state—the holistic sensation that people feel when they act with total involve-

ment—as *flow*. In the flow state, action follows upon action according to an internal logic that seems to need no conscious intervention by the actor. He experiences it as a unified flowing from one moment to the next, in which he is in control of his actions, and in which there is little distinction between self and environment, between stimulus and response, between past, present, and future.[52]

As Csikszentmihalyi's study progressed, he saw that while flow activities were often related to games and play, they were also the key elements in other activities, such as creativity, love, and what are usually called religious, or transcendental, or "peak experiences": "In a variety of human contexts, then, one finds a remarkably similar inner state, which is so enjoyable that people are sometimes willing to forsake a comfortable life for its sake." With this remarkable insight, Csikszentmihalvi unites games, play, creativity, love, and religion as things that are "enjoyable" by means of giving us "flow."

He then proceeds to enumerate what he has discovered to be the essential elements of all flow experiences: The first is the "merging of action and awareness." "For flow to be maintained," the professor says, "one cannot reflect on the act of awareness itself. When awareness becomes split, so that one perceives the activity from 'outside,' flow is interrupted.... These interruptions occur when questions flash through the actor's mind: 'Am I doing well?' 'What am I doing here?' ... When one is in a flow episode ... these questions simply do not come to mind."

People who have experienced flow would like to be able to control it—to be able to make it happen when they want it to. Unfortunately, flow is quite elusive. That's why, when people find some activity that allows them frequently to enter a flow state, they become "addicts" of that state. They have found something that works for them, and they are loath to change it. One reason flow is so elusive, according to Csikszentmihalyi, is that the difficulty of the activity must be perfectly matched to the abilities of the practitioner. He illustrates this by describing all activities as lying on a spectrum: At one end the activities present no challenges or difficulties at all, and at the other end they pose such extraordinary challenges that they're far beyond the capabilities of the practitioner. At one end of the spectrum is boredom; at the other end, anxiety.

This necessity of an even match between the difficulty of a challenge and a person's ability to meet it shows why the most common experiences of flow occur in games, rituals, participatory art and athletic forms like dance and sports, and in activities with clear rules governing the action. In such activities the participants can control the level of difficulty or adjust the level of challenge to meet their skills—unlike "real life," where the rules and the level of difficulty are beyond the control of most of us. A group of eight-year-olds can experience as much pure pleasure and flow from their game of pickup baseball on the corner lot as can the much more highly skilled major league superstars; a golfer can adjust his handicap; a marathoner an hour behind the winners is challenging his personal best.

This brings us to the float tank. In the preceding summary, floaters will quickly have recognized an exact description of the float experience. The essential qualities of flow—a sense of discovery, exploration, problem solution, novelty, challenge, merging of action and awareness, timelessness, a sense of control emerging from a perfect matching of difficulty with ability, and above all the feeling of great pleasure that results from the combination of these elements—are also the essential qualities of floating. Even the word *flow* is evocative of the tank experience.

A key fact that Dr. Csikszentmihalyi emphasizes again and again is that in everyday life, flow experiences are elusive. Even in game or play situations expressly designed to elicit them, they are often lacking, or are experienced only for fleeting moments that emerge unexpectedly and unpredictably between longer periods of more mundane concerns. It is here that we see the unique value of floating: The floatation tank is a specific and reliable flow-creation tool. On the whole, floaters seem to experience flow every time they enter the tank. Even better, they experience that most elusive and pleasurable thing, long periods of pure, uninterrupted flow.

One reason the tank has this unique effect is that it is both *experience and environment.* The rock climber must go to the mountain; the chess player must find the perfectly matched opponent; the athlete waits for the ideal moment in the contest to draw him beyond his own limits. But for the floater both the experience and the environment are right there, any time, in the tank. As for the matching of challenge with ability, there is no need to find the consummate opponent or teammates or situation: the floater can adjust the inherent difficulty or challenge of both the experience and the environment so that they perfectly match and make full use of his or her skills, whether it's the first time in the tank or the fifty-first. When you float, there is nothing happening in the tank that is not you. That is, everything that goes on in the tank is either what you "do" or what you "don't do." In Dr. Lilly's words, *"Nothing can happen that you will not allow to happen, i.e.: what is forbidden is not allowed."* [139]

Another explanation for the tank's unique effect is that it seems to operate specifically by eliminating both boredom and anxiety. There is much physiological and psychological evidence that in the tank the floater's mind remains extraordinarily alert, and alertness seems to counteract all boredom by involving us deeply in our awareness. When the alert mind is lodged in the relaxed body fostered by floating, you have a combination particularly conducive to the experience of flow.

Narrowing the Field of Consciousness.   Another absolute necessity for attaining the flow experience is what Dr. Csikszentmihalyi describes as "a centering of attention on a limited stimulus field. To ensure that people will concentrate on their actions, potentially intruding stimuli must be kept out of attention." Many people find that this is a natural consequence of the merging of awareness and activity: "I got so wrapped up in playing that game that I didn't even hear you talking to me." Games, rituals, and the like also help narrow the field of consciousness by controlling the environment.

Floatation tanks are particularly effective in this narrowing of consciousness, since they not only focus the floater's attention on the moment, but actually restrict, through physical means, the external stimuli that can often distract someone from the flow experience. Noises, light, other people, unexpected events, and much more are eliminated by the tank itself.

Increased Awareness.   Csikszentmihalyi insists, however, that the narrowing of consciousness of the flow experience does not mean one loses touch with one's own physical reality. Rather, "one becomes more intensely aware of internal processes." He notes the increased muscular awareness of rock climbers, and chess players' exquisite awareness of the workings of their own minds, and concludes: "What is usually lost in flow is not the awareness of one's body or of one's functions, but only the *self construct*, the intermediary which one learns to interpose between stimulus and response."

This observation rings true to floaters, since one of the most obvious effects of floating is increased physical awareness (see Feldenkrais's discussion of the Weber-Fechner Law on page 48). In fact, many floaters use the tank for exactly this reason: as a powerful tool for changing behavior, breaking habits, and improving their state of health.

The Experience of Control.   An important characteristic of the person in flow is his control of himself and his environment. As Csikszentmihalyi observes, "He has no active awareness of control but is simply not worried by the possibility of lack of control. Later, in thinking back on the experience, he will usually conclude that, for the duration of the experience, his skills were adequate for meeting environmental demands; and this reflection might become an important component of a positive self-concept."[52]

We've already observed that the floatation tank is a completely controllable environment, but the idea that the feeling of control and competence one gets from floating can lead to a positive self-concept is very important. Therapists have long recognized the feeling of control as an important component of self-confidence and self-esteem. It is partly because of this feeling of control, and the resulting increase in self confidence and self-esteem, that floatation has had such powerfully beneficial effects on people suffering from depression, anxiety, self destructive tendencies, and lack of confidence. Interestingly, there is a biochemical component to increased control. Recent studies show that while elevated levels of cortisol are linked to feelings of submission, reduced levels of cortisol are linked to feelings of confidence and dominance. As we have seen, floating has been shown to decrease cortisol levels significantly.

One example of heightened self-esteem through floating is Chris, the model haunted by a rape attempt. When she went into the tank she discovered to her pleasure that she felt she could control what happened to her. She felt like an explorer who was continually making successful voyages of discovery. As she said to me: "Every time I float I feel like an adventurer, and I'm proud of myself." Nothing succeeds like success; or, success comes easier to those who are used to conquering. And those who have experienced the sense of competence and control that comes from floating are able to transfer it and continue to experience it in their everyday lives.

Dr. Csikszentmihalyi observes that the feeling of control we have in flow is difficult to sustain for any length of time in the real world, where things are always somewhat beyond control. However, it has become clear that it's possible to train yourself to carry the feeling of control—that is, flow—with you into your everyday life.

Flowing on the Subway. I can personally attest to how the float, and flow, experience can be carried into the real world. I had been working one afternoon in midtown Manhattan and by the time I descended into the subway to go home it was exactly 5:00 P.M. The Times Square train was packed so full with rush-hour riders that it was impossible to raise a hand or even to move. The train was midway to the 34th Street station when it suddenly stopped, the motors shut down with a cough and were silent, and all the lights went out, inspiring screams from many of the passengers. As the situation became clear, a wave of moans swept through the train. If the temperature in the streets had been 95 degrees, it was more than 110 in the subway; the air conditioner was shut off, the windows were sealed, and we were all crammed together, sweating and blind in the dark. I heard gasps and felt shudders of panic from the stranger pressed against me, and the motorman's voice came over the loudspeaker telling us that some insane person had jumped on the tracks at Penn Station and the police were trying to get him off. Since the man was holding his foot next to the third rail, the electricity had been shut off, and we had no choice but to sit there sweltering in the dark until the juice was turned back on. It was apparent to all of us that this could take some time. Several people yelled that they were having trouble breathing. Someone shouted a suggestion to break the windows while others shouted not to break the windows. People nearby began screaming that an old man was having a heart attack.

While I'm not claustrophobic, I felt myself growing very tense. I had an instinctive desire to move, to get out of there, but not only was there no room to run, there was no room to move at all. I had a powerful sense that this was a situation over which I had no control. I felt my chest constrict and my muscles tighten. The woman behind me began to sob loudly. Then I remembered the experience of the floatation tank: I had been floating a few days earlier, and as I thought of the deeply peaceful relaxation of the tank, it was as if my body actually remembered how it felt to be there. I made a conscious effort to imagine I was in the tank, and felt all my muscles relax, my breathing grow, deep and easy. Calm and peace took hold, and I even experienced my external situation of being trapped in the dark train as blackly funny. I envisioned my explanation to the person I was supposed to meet at five, and how she would scoff at my lame excuse. The train was stuck for almost an hour, and I felt a sense of flow the whole time. A small thing, but for me it was a clear sign of how the floating experience can be carried over into the less controllable real world, and how the experience of floating can be effective training for experiencing flow in the daily routine.

Dr. Csikszentmihalyi seems to be referring to something like this when he says, "Ideally, anyone could learn to carry inside himself the tools of enjoyment. But whether the structure is internal or external, the steps for experiencing flow are presumably the same; they involve the same process of delimiting reality, controlling some aspects of it, and responding to the feedback with a concentration that excludes anything else as irrelevant." Once again, it seems that floating and flow are identical.

Intrinsic Rewards. Like all flow experiences, the rewards of floating can be found in the experience itself. Some perceive the floatation tank, with its intrinsic rewards, as being inherently selfish or escapist, a product of the "Me Generation." We must make the world a better place, they argue, rather than retreating into ourselves.

Csikszentmihalyi addresses this common misperception movingly:

> In this society, where the opportunity to satisfy pleasure and to obtain material comforts is unprecedented, the statistics on crime, mental disease, alcoholism, venereal disease, gambling, dissatisfaction with work, drug abuse, and general discontent keep steadily worsening. The rates of these indices of alienation are increasing more sharply in the affluent suburbs. It is not the bottling up of instinctual needs that is responsible for this trend, nor the lack of external rewards. Its cause appears to be the dearth of experiences which prove that one is competent, in a system that is geared for the efficient transformation of physical energy. The lack of intrinsic rewards is like an undiscovered virus we carry in our bodies; it maims slowly but surely.[52]

Someone who has been able to develop his ability to flow at will, or to "resonate his abilities with the environment," is in harmony with his world. Csikszentmihalyi stresses that one could be in solitary confinement or in a boring job, but if he knows how to respond to this environment with flow, he will still experience enjoyment, and such a person "becomes both truly autonomous and truly connected with the world. Extrinsic rewards will be less needed to motivate him to put up with the hardships of existence. A constant ability to 'design or discover something new,' 'to explore a strange place'—the rewards that people experience in deep flow—will be enough to motivate action. Only with such a shift in perspective will we avoid 'devouring the world.' We must 'deliberately choose a life of action over a life of consumption,' or the human and physical resources of our environment will be depleted."

The flow experience, then, is not self-indulgent, selfish, antisocial. On the contrary, it is the person who has learned to experience flow, through the training of numerous flow experiences such as those acquired in the floatation tank, who is in the forefront of social evolution. Flow is not an escape from life but life lived at a higher level.

FOURTEEN

THE AQUATIC APE
EXPLANATION

Is the float tank experience a sort of return to the womb? A lot of people think so. The idea is so widespread that one commercial float center is called The Womb Room. The parallels are striking: floating in dense warm salt solution, in a dark, secure, enclosed space; theta brain waves (like those of babies) creating a sense of timelessness; a dim awareness that at some uncertain future time one will have to emerge from this safe haven into a different, less peaceful place ....

Preliminary studies by Fine and Turner of the Medical College of Ohio, suggesting that floating causes an increased secretion of the body's natural narcotics, endorphins,[252] take on an intriguing significance when considered in this light. Endorphins are released from the pituitary gland, and it's known that pregnant women develop an extra lobe of the pituitary gland. Tests have also shown that pregnant women have up to eight times the normal amount of endorphins in their blood. These endorphins flow freely across the placenta during pregnancy, so the fetus is also experiencing an extraordinarily high level of endorphins. In fact, endorphins seem to be a literal mother substitute. When puppies, chicks, and young guinea pigs that had been separated from their mothers were given doses of endorphins, they stopped crying and ceased to experience stress. The neuroscientist conducting the experiment remarked, "Almost as if opiates are neurochemically equivalent to the presence of mother, the animals given endorphins were quickly comforted."[101]

Endorphins not only relieve pain; like the other opiates, such as heroin and morphine, they create states of intense euphoria. Prenatal bliss, then, is a physiologically real experience; probably the prototypical high to which all our other joys and experiences are compared and found sadly wanting. So when we're suspended in the warm dark tank, body pulsing rhythmically with an audible and reassuring heart beat, with our brains pumping out endorphins, it's quite possible some subconscious memory is stirred and profoundly deep emotional associations called up.

Mommy and I Are One.   These speculations become even more interesting when we consider recent research in subliminal perception done by Lloyd Silverman. Silverman was originally interested in using subliminal perception to desensitize people who had fear of cockroaches. Using the tachitoscope, a special machine that flashes a message faster than a viewer can consciously see it, he flashed the neutral message "People are walking" to one group. To the other group, he flashed the loaded message "Mommy and I are one." After four sessions, the group which had subliminally seen "Mommy and I are one" had made far more improvement than the control group.

Silverman then used the same technique to improve academic performance. Law students, all evenly matched academically before the study, were randomly assigned to two groups and shown the two different subliminal messages four times a week over a six-week summer session. At the end the Mommy group received substantially higher grades than the other group. Silverman concluded that the power of the Mommy message was as a "magical fulfillment of ... wishes emanating from the earliest developmental level, particularly wishes for oral gratification and maternal warmth."[217,218]

Psychologist and author Howard Halpern observes of these fascinating results that the Mommy message seemed to act as "insurance that Mother won't leave and abandon them, and a reduction in the threat they experience in temporary separations because, after all, Mommy and I are one; and a fusion with Mother's strength can magically remedy all shortcomings and impairments."[93] In their book about these experiments, *The Search for Oneness*, Silverman and his associates go on to discuss how this pursuit for fusion with Mommy, the search for oneness, can become the most powerful impulse in life, impelling people to such varied pursuits as meditation, religious experiences of all sorts, drugs and alcohol, religious cults, and jogging.[218]

If the need for oneness, for fusion with Mother's strength, is so powerful, and the float tank is such a striking and convincing analogue of the womb, then we have compelling answers to why the tank is such a satisfying and confidence-building experience, and why people who float often feel that their lives take on wholeness. If an hour or two of floating in the tank can provide us with an intense experience of the oneness that is the essential pursuit of our lives, then we have an explanation for floaters' frequent spontaneous reduction in fears, spontaneous reduction in smoking, drinking, and drug taking, and a noticeable influx of energy, creativity, and productivity into their lives.

The Floating Ape

The womb hypothesis is interesting, but maybe we're not taking a long range view of the satisfying sense of "Ah, home at last" that so many feel on entering the tank. Returning to the womb is a return over only a few years of a single individual's life. It is also possible that the return is one of several million years, to the earliest days of the evolution of our species, when, as anthropologists now believe, for a period of hundreds of thousands and perhaps millions of years, early humans lived as aquatic or semiaquatic creatures, gathering shellfish and living in the shallows of great inland seas.

The aquatic theory was first advanced by the British biologist of aquatic life Sir Alistair Hardy, and has gained a considerable following in recent years. Among the most prominent proponents of the hypothesis is Elaine Morgan, who recently devoted an entire volume to exploring it (*The Aquatic Ape: A Theory of Human Evolution*). Morgan cites recent geological and anthropological evidence that a crucial gap in human fossil history (the yawning gap between the very ape-like and knuckle-walking *Ramapithecus*, whose fossils are dated around 9 million years ago, and *Australopithecus*, who walked upright on two legs and whose foot imprints are almost exactly like ours, whose fossil remains date from about 3.7 million years ago), coincided with a time when large areas of Africa were flooded and covered by vast seas, with the exception of some large upland areas that became islands. Morgan explains:

> The aquatic theory envisages that during this period one group of apes embarked on a distinct path of evolution by adapting to an aquatic environment—just as other species had done earlier [e.g. dolphins, whales, porpoises, all warm-blooded mammals whose skeletons show the remnants of legs, indicating they once lived on land before returning to the sea]. Later, when the waters receded and new ecological opportunities opened up, they returned to their former terrestrial lifestyle. But they brought with them a package of in-built aquatic adaptations, which they still demonstrably retain.... The theory suggests that man did not lose his hair because he became an overheated hunter.... He lost it for the same reason as the whale and the dolphin and the manatee: because if any fairly large aquatic mammal needs to keep warm in water, it is better served by a layer of fat on the inside of its skin than by a layer of hair on the outside of it.[168]

In her ingenious and fascinating treatise, Morgan shows how satisfactorily the aquatic theory explains many otherwise inexplicable points of human nature and physiology. For example, to adapt to life in the water, early humans developed the ability to close the nasal passages and throat, and to hold their breath for deep diving (a skill other primates—who are afraid of the water—do not have). In developing the soft palate and unique throat structure and nasal cavity, humans also developed the ability to enunciate words (other primates are physiologically unable to do so), out of which came our speech and other verbal abilities. The theory also explains the recent discovery that babies are able to swim not merely before they're able to walk but even before they can crawl. Not only do babies have a swimming reflex, but breath-holding and diving reflexes as well. The theory also explains why humans weep salt tears, copulate face to face, have no body hair, walk on two legs rather than knuckle-walking like our ape cousins, and have developed such a large neocortex.

Does this theory hold water? Throw it in the lake and see if it floats. If it has any validity (and both Morgan and Hardy produce persuasive arguments), then we are water babies in more ways than one and salt water is our natural element, the evolutionary matrix of our species for as many as 5 million years. We were made to float; it's in our genes. Buoyant basking beasts. And each time we lie back on the supportive salt water, bobbing blissfully, our breath booming rhythmically in our ears like surf, we are connecting with our heritage, stirring our cellular memory, communing with some ancient self—that primordial Australopithecan cousin, floating pensively in the warm, shallow salt sea of northern Africa 5 million years back, humming and burbling soulfully with our delightful and unique vocal tract and resonant nasal passages, and preparing to crack open a succulent shellfish on our hairless belly with a rock. O brave new world, that has such people in it!

FIFTEEN

THE HOMEOSTASIS EXPLANATION

In many of these "explanations" of floatation we have been dealing with the nebulous borderline between mind and body. The singular experience of floating in an enclosed tank does certain measurable things to your body, which in turn influences your state of mind; likewise, the tank experience has noticeable effects on your state of mind, which can produce numerous changes in your body. Which comes first? The answer to this chicken and egg problem, of course, is that neither exists without the other; they are not separate systems at all, but one system, united in a relationship of balance and interaction.

The first scientist to develop a convincing model of this interaction between psyche and soma was Walter B. Cannon, of Harvard Medical School, in his influential book *The Wisdom of the Body*, published in 1932.[44] One of Cannon's central ideas was that the body has an inherent "wisdom," which consists of an exquisitely sensitive self-monitoring and self-regulating system centered in the hypothalamus that is constantly working to maintain the body in an optimal state of balance, harmony, equilibrium, stability. This optimal state, in which all parts and systems are interacting properly, is called *homeostasis*.

Since the body is always changing, and having to deal with changing conditions, any mechanism to keep the body in equilibrium must be able to maintain stability in the midst of flux, must respond with infinite adaptability to a constantly changing environment. Think of trying to carry a full cup of hot coffee across the rolling deck of a storm-tossed ship—what is required is flexibility and the ability to accommodate one's direction and attitude to any sudden alteration in the environment. In other words, homeostasis is relative: a *process* rather than a predetermined state. If we placed a subject in icy water, we might conclude that the body maintained homeostasis by keeping the body temperature very high. But if we placed that same subject in a sauna, we would have to conclude that homeostasis involved various mechanisms such as sweating that let the body disperse heat. Homeostasis, however, is neither "keeping body temperature high" nor "dispersing body heat"; it is the mechanism that responds to heat, cold, or any other conditions the body might have to operate under.

This marvelous instinctual maintenance of the integrity of the whole human system has been compared to a series of feedback loops. Like the simple house thermostat that turns off when the temperature reaches a certain level and switches on when the temperature falls below another level, the body is constantly monitoring and responding to body temperatures, levels of blood sugar, oxygen, salt, and so on. The most refined examples of biological homeostasis are the exquisitely sensitive feedback loops of the endocrine system. The main control center of the endocrine system is the hypothalamus, which ceaselessly tests the level of numerous chemicals in the blood and responds to any imbalance by signaling the pituitary to secrete hormones to correct it.

Within this section we have briefly explored a number of quite different approaches to floating. While each successfully "explains" some of the remarkable effects of floating, none of them purports to offer an overriding theory, a superordinate explanation of exactly how and why floating works. None of these explanations, that is, is *the* explanation. However, when we see them not as competing theories but rather as integral parts of a single system—parts that interact synergistically, dynamically, to create a whole that is greater than the sum of the parts — we begin to perceive the real nature of the unified-field theory of floating. Taken together, I think these various explanations constitute a sort of body, with its own type of homeostasis.

Homeostasis and Stress. The concept of homeostasis offers not just a way of looking at the relationship among the various approaches to a study of floating; homeostasis is in fact the underlying factor in all the explanations, an inwoven thread uniting each of the explanations. In The Relaxation Response Explanation, for example, we saw how floating can counteract a pathological arousal of the sympathetic nervous system by bringing into play a balancing, compensatory force, the parasympathetic response. Stress is seen as the external influence that the body must respond to, the relaxation response as the force which maintains or restores homeostasis.

Like all homeostatic mechanisms, however, the relaxation response is not good *in itself,* but only as a means of maintaining the body's optimal state. As with blood sugar or adrenaline, too much is just as harmful as too little, and excessive dominance of the parasympathetic system can manifest itself as, for example, pathological depression. Phil Nuernberger, director of biofeedback therapy at the Minneapolis Clinic of Psychiatry and Neurology, calls this overdominance of parasympathetic activity The Possum Response. When faced with a threatening situation, people who have an overactive parasympathetic response don't prepare to fight or run away; "they just sort of roll over and play dead. Their response to fear is not arousal, but inhibition. This is marked by the typical characteristics of extreme parasympathetic discharge—decreased physiological functioning, loss of skeletal tone, mental lassitude, inactivity, and eventual depression." [173] As Nuernberger points out, this imbalance can be as harmful as chronic hyperarousal of the fight-or-flight response. Depression is a causative factor in many illnesses. That is, the helplessness and hopelessness of depression can be just as stressful as chronic hyperarousal.

This brings us to an interesting view of stress: Rather than considering it simply as a hyperarousal of our fight-or-flight response, it is better understood as a *state of unbalance,* a disruption of our internal equilibrium—that is, a disturbance of our homeostasis. And the theory of stress as *interruption,* discussed earlier—that stress results from discrepancies between expectations and reality—can now be seen as a psychological equivalent of the *disruption* of homeostasis. Homeostasis is what our body "expects," it is the norm; when this norm is interrupted, when the world of our body becomes not the way it was, then we experience stress.

In the case of the sympathetic and parasympathetic responses, the floatation tank seems to counteract stress by maintaining homeostasis. As we saw in the chapter on flow, one characteristic of floating is that it tends to increase the floater's sense of confidence, capability, and power. That is, it seems to help people overcome depression by counteracting their excessive parasympathetic or possum response. It also seems to work against overactivation of the parasympathetic response by causing the body to release certain natural antidepressant and euphoria-causing neurochemicals, such as the endorphins. At the same time, floating powerfully reduces overactivation of the sympathetic, fight-or-flight response. Floatation seems to work not simply as a consistent counterbalance to the fight-or-flight response on the one hand, or to the possum response on the other, but as a balancing force between both—a maintainer of homeostasis.

This same observation holds true in many other of the explanations I have offered. We saw that floatation tends to work on our chronic imbalance between right hemisphere and left, not by simply shifting the dominance to the minor hemisphere but by bringing the imbalanced right and left hemispheres into a state of symmetry and synchrony in which the entire apparatus of the brain is unified and works in harmony—that is, hemispheric homeostasis.

While not enough research has been done yet on the effects of floatation on our biochemicals, what we do know indicates that floating's beneficial effects can be attributed not to some constant and unvarying relationship between floating and, say, serotonin, but to its power in allowing the body to establish a homeostatic balance. Medical researchers Fine and Turner of the Medical College of Ohio reached a similar conclusion when trying to understand how short periods of floatation could have such significant long-term effects on numerous hormones and other body functions such as blood pressure. "In light of the carry-over effect" of the floating on the hormone levels, they concluded that repeated floating "could alter the set-points or baselines of the endocrine homeostatic mechanisms." [252]

Homeostasis seems to be the principle at work in most of the observed effects of floating. Even things like spontaneous reduction in smoking or addictive behavior can be seen as the body's natural tendency to restore itself to its optimal state.

Why is the tank so effective in fostering homeostasis? If we see the mind/body as a single system, then it becomes clear that external stimuli are constantly militating against the system's equilibrium: Every noise, every degree of temperature above or below the body's optimal level, every encounter with other people, every feeling of responsibility, guilt, desire—everything we see and feel is incessantly interrupting, impinging on our self-contained system, causing it to expend energy to maintain its homeostatic balance. But when we enter the tank, our environment abruptly stops its constant alteration. The system is for once able to experience itself as a single, integral, unified entity. Since there are no external threats, no need to adapt to outside events, no deviations from the expected, the system can devote all its energies to restoring itself. It is as if we said *Time out* to the game of life, allowing our bodies to take a breather and restore themselves to normal. The normal state, of course, is health, vigor, enthusiasm, and immense pleasure in being alive. The way the body gets there, and stays there, is homeostasis.

PART III

WAYS OF FLOATING

Every type of crucial experiment proves that what we see and where we see it, depends entirely upon the physiological functioning of our body. Any method of making our body function internally in a given way, will provide us with an assigned visual sensation. The body is supremely indifferent to the happenings of nature a short way off, where it places its visual sensa.

Now the same is true of all other modes of sensation, only to a greater extent. All sense-perception is merely one outcome of the dependence of our experience upon bodily functioning. Thus if we wish to understand the relation of our personal experience to the activities of nature, the proper procedure is to examine the dependence of our personal experiences upon our personal bodies.

—ALFRED NORTH WHITEHEAD, ***Modes of Thought***

SIXTEEN

DEEP RELAXATION
AND BEYOND

"I was desperately trying to clear all these thoughts out of my head and relax." Alice, a commercial artist who had had much experience in meditation before her first float, was describing her experience in the tank. "I was meditating, counting breaths, trying everything, but I couldn't seem to get relaxed, or quiet down my mind. After about forty minutes I thought, *Well, I guess I'm just not going to be able to relax this time. Forget it.* And as soon as I let go, and stopped trying, it was like everything fell away and there I was—you know, THERE— and I thought to myself, *Well, here I am.*"

Alice's experience is quite common and instructive. A major reason for the floatation tank's extraordinary range of effects is that, while floating, our bodies become more deeply relaxed than is possible in every day life, and this happens effortlessly. But it's essential to remember that *effortless* means exactly that—efforts we make in the tank will only hinder our relaxation, and that includes efforts to relax. Alice went into the tank with great expectations, but found that it was only when she reached a point of letting go that she was actually able to relax; that in the tank she could only do things by not doing, create by giving up creative intentions, get someplace by deciding not to go anyplace at all.

It's a phenomenon humans have been aware of ever since they started paying attention to how their minds worked, but—as seems necessary in this technological age—one that has recently been quantified and demonstrated with sensitive electronic equipment in the labs of scientists studying the methods and effects of biofeedback. They have found the phenomenon so predictable and regular that they've incorporated it into training programs as lesson number one and given it a name: The Law of Reversed Effort. Whatever you "try" to do, the result will be just the opposite.

There is a certain trick to letting go but it is quite easy to learn, and once learned it's not easily forgotten. One of the most momentous discoveries of the biofeedback wave was finding out that a person who has experienced and learned to identify a certain internal state can then control and re-create that internal state at will. The floatation tank is a natural biofeedback tool that works in part by permitting us to become aware of subtle and minute internal changes and states, among them deep relaxation. And for first-time floaters the experience is much like being hooked up to a biofeedback machine for the first time: The harder they try to achieve the desired state, the more it escapes them, until finally they learn—almost by accident—to let go, and the state just happens. Like biofeedback machine users, floaters soon master the trick of letting go. Many speak of having a "body memory" of it, and most learn to let themselves sink into the familiar state of deep relaxation within minutes after getting into the tank.

Brain research now suggests that everything we ever experience is stored away in the brain somewhere and can be instantly recalled if we know the right signal. Clearly the state of deep relaxation is stored away in the mind, so that at any moment we can call it up out of our gray matter and experience it fully again. This is accomplished by giving the body a signal that identifies and locates the specific mind/body configuration, so that the mind can retrieve it from its storage system.

One example of the body's recall of deep relaxation is my experience on the stalled subway, when my body seemed to remember the blackness, silence, warmth, smell, and total muscular relaxation of the tank. The effect was like a click—one moment tension, then suddenly everything fell into place. Another example of just how real this body memory is, and how it can respond to a signal, was revealed by Arthur, the chess-playing psychologist, who told me that since he began floating he had found that each morning's warm bath water seemed to put him right back into the serene mood he felt in the tank. "I guess you could say it's a conditioned reflex," he said, "but that bath makes me feel like I have everything under control, and what's amazing is that I carry this feeling with me throughout the day. It's as if my morning bath were a kind of 'little float,' reminding my body of the real float."

Once you have entered this state of profound relaxation, and learned to reenter it and maintain it effortlessly, you find that it is an ideal state in which to utilize any of a wide range of techniques for behavior or attitude change: self-hypnosis, autosuggestion, visualization, free-flowing imagery, self-healing, prayer, meditation, autogenics exercises, and so on. Controlled studies at several universities in which floaters were compared with people using other deep relaxation and behavior modification techniques, including meditation, autogenics, progressive relaxation, autosuggestion, and guided imagery, have demonstrated that *all methods of mental or physical self-regulation or self-control work more powerfully and effectively in the floatation tank than in any other environment.*

The essential element common to all such techniques is that the subject must be in a state of deep relaxation. The environment of the tank is unsurpassed for attaining and maintaining relaxation, and virtually everyone who goes into the tank will reach a state of deep relaxation sooner or later.

But beginning or inexperienced floaters should remember that the best strategy to take when going into the tank is no strategy at all. The floaters I've talked with agree: For the first few floats don't set any goals. Says neuroendocrinologist John Turner, who has conducted float research on hundreds of subjects: "We've found that novice floaters usually need to float four or five times before they really begin to get in touch." On the other hand, just about everyone agrees that the first or second float is the most fun, the most mind-boggling. So lie back, allow your subconscious to choose what *it* wants to deal with, and let your body find its own path to deep relaxation. If you have no expectations, you will never be disappointed.

Ways of Letting Go
Having issued this dictum against effort of any sort, let me immediately contradict myself by saying that there are a number of techniques that floaters have found helpful in reaching states of ultra-deep relaxation. Actually there's no real contradiction, since my initial point is that deep relaxation is a state most novice floaters will not have tasted before, and since they have no prior experience of it they will not be able to find their way there by means of conscious effort. However, *after* we've become accustomed to the tank environment, have experienced deep relaxation, then it is quite possible to return to that state quickly, either in the tank or outside it when we want to draw on body memory of the floating state. This rapid return to deep relaxation can be facilitated by certain methods or techniques, some of them familiar to initiates of meditation and other self-regulation or mind-control practices. But using these techniques in the tank is different, not only in degree but in quality. For one thing, they are much more effective in the tank, and can carry you more rapidly to a much deeper state than you may have experienced before. Following are some of the techniques that experienced floaters have found particularly effective in the tank.

Breath Awareness. An effective method of freeing the body from the interference of the conscious mind, and of stilling the distracting flow of thoughts, images, and words through the mind, is to focus your attention on your breathing. Since all other senses have been restricted, and ears are submerged, the sounds of your body can take on monumental proportions: Your lungs can become huge bellows, your breath a wind howling through a vast cavern, a manifestation of the basic dualistic pulse of life, forces flowing in/out.

Abdominal Breathing.   It's essential to relax your abdominal muscles, so that when you inhale, your belly expands and rises. Many people believe they'll look unattractive that way, and so they maintain a constant tension in their bellies, wasting energy and hampering their ability to breathe fully. Instead of breathing by expanding and contracting the diaphragm and belly, they expand and contract the chest and rib cage. This shallow breathing uses only the top part of the lungs, and more important, it is one of the physiological correlates of the tight-or-flight reaction. Thus, by breathing in our chests, we cause our autonomic nervous systems to maintain a constant condition of arousal, adding to the stress to which our systems are subjected.

Nose Breathing.   A popular breathing practice among floaters is simply to focus the attention on the breath as it passes in and out of the nose. Feel the air pass into your nostrils as you inhale; focus on the coolness it brings to the tip of your nose between your nostrils. As you exhale, notice the warmth at the same spot. If you wish, count your inhalations, numbering each from one to ten; when you reach ten begin with one again. Should thoughts come into your awareness, don't resist them but allow them to pass, and then return all attention to your breathing.

Moving Around the Body.   This technique effectively combines breathing awareness and rhythm with focused awareness of various parts of the body. With each breath, count a number and direct your total attention to a particular spot in your body; feel as if your entire being is in that spot. On the count of one, place your attention in the center of your forehead. With the second breath, count two and concentrate on your throat. With three, move to your right shoulder. Then, with succeeding counts, move down your right arm (elbow, wrist, each finger) and back up the arm to the throat. Do the same with your left arm. Next move to your chest, abdomen, pelvis, then down your right leg (hip, knee, ankle, each toe), back up the leg, across the pelvis, and down your left leg. Return to your abdomen and move back upward, ending at your forehead again. Depending on your exact route, this should take about sixty breaths. You will find that as your attention moves from place to place, it creates, and is accompanied by, very definite body sensations. In my own experience, each part of the body that I count becomes quite warm and, in my mind's eye, seems to glow with warm white light as it noticeably releases tension, "melts," grows "softer" and more relaxed. The entire sequence takes only a few minutes, but by the time you have returned to the center of your forehead you will be deeply relaxed. (This has been adapted from a technique of Swami Rama, and Elmer and Alyce Green.)

Practicing Visualization
Anyone can profit from improving his or her ability to visualize, but those whose mental imagery is weak or undeveloped, the people who really need the most practice, are the ones most likely to avoid it, like non-swimmers who simply stay out of the water. These people especially can find the float tank the ideal environment for visualization practice; while it is improving the vividness of mental imagery, it also eliminates the presence of other people who may inspire feelings of competitiveness or pressure, and, since researchers have found that poor visualizers often combine a low opinion of "daydreaming" with a rigid "dictatorship of the will" (in the words of psychologist Robert Sommer),[224] the float tank provides an excuse for daydreaming. There's nothing else to do in there. A number of strongly verbal people I've spoken to who float regularly—lawyers, a salesman, a philosophy professor—take an almost childlike delight in their newfound ability to manipulate mental images in the tank. They think it has given them new awareness of the other people they deal with in life, as well as opening them up to previously untapped energies and ideas.

Body Imagery. What we see in the mind's eye has a decided influence over our physical and mental states, and an excellent way of practicing visualization is to combine imagery with floating's intense sensory awareness for the purpose of deepening one's level of relaxation. For example, the nose-breathing exercise mentioned above can be combined with imagery to increase its power: Visualize the air entering your nostrils as pure white light. As you inhale, follow the flow of white light through your nasal passages, into your lungs, into your abdomen; visualize the light in your belly, pulsing, radiating to every part of your body. Then, as you exhale, see the light flow back out of your body. Focus on your breathing entirely.

Visualization of Light. As, breathing, you see the light pouring into your body, pure, white or golden, bearing oxygen and life energy, radiant, vibrating, glowing, envision its life-enhancing force spreading through your body. Then, as you breathe out, visualize the energy as dark blue, or gray, or brown—it is now filled with waste material, toxins, fatigue, distortions, which it is carrying out of your system. As you continue to inhale energy, exhale waste, visualize your entire body growing brighter, full of glowing vitality, glowing so brightly the entire inside of the tank is filled with dazzling light. Try variations, such as seeing your bones glowing with blinding light, or your blood vessels pulsing with sparkling energy.

Moving Light Around the Body.   Another variation of this is to use it with the exercise in which you count as you move from point to point around the body. With each count, as you focus your center of attention on another spot, see that spot glowing warmly, with a golden light. This will enhance the relaxing, centering effect of this exercise.

In the Mind's Eye.   Another way to strengthen your control of imagery (and, as a result, of your body) is consciously to manipulate colors and images not associated with your body. For example, as you float, imagine a box of paints or crayons. See each color. How do these colors affect you? Visualize various shapes: a cube, a sphere, a pyramid. See a bright red sphere against a green backdrop; then change the colors. Try a familiar cartoon figure: See Mickey Mouse, Roadrunner, Pinocchio, Fred Flintstone. Visualize them running, or dancing. Create a scene for them. Watch a figure dancing before you; see it talking to you as if you were a camera recording its performance. What is the figure saying?

Imagine yourself in a familiar scene, perhaps the bedroom you slept in as a child. See it clearly; notice the furniture, objects placed about the room. What does this scene make you feel? Now rearrange it somehow: Put a piano in the room, or a gorilla. Visualize yourself walking around the room, looking at all the furniture from different angles. Introduce someone into the room who was never there—your spouse, your office rival. What do you feel when you combine these images'?

Visualize someone you know well: See the face; notice the texture of the skin, the color of the eyes; see how the face is changed by a smile. Now see that person moving, perhaps dancing or gesturing to you.

Watch as the person speaks to you; see the eyes focused on you and hear the voice. What is being said to you? Pay attention; it is probably something important.

Visualize yourself, your face. Smile at yourself. Observe carefully. Notice everything. What clothes are you wearing? Is there something about you that you don't like? Now visualize yourself doing something—playing tennis perhaps, or climbing a mountain. What are you doing? See yourself laughing. Now the image is speaking to you. What are you saying to yourself?

Now that you can see yourself, envision yourself very large. You are like Gulliver among the Lilliputians, towering over buildings. Now very small. Like the Incredible Shrinking Man, make yourself as small as a cell, an atom. You might want to enter your own body and move through your system— check up on your kidneys, boat down the alimentary canal.

Practice of these visualization techniques is fun, and will reveal to you in a very direct way exactly what's on your mind. Often it will surprise you. These visualizations are also the foundation for healing and self-regulatory techniques described in later chapters.

SEVENTEEN

BEYOND RELAXATION—
SELF-HYPNOSIS

I'd been floating for about an hour, and several times had focused on my right foot, trying to tune in to the problem there. I had succeeded in getting rid of the pain, but every time I turned my attention elsewhere, I was brought back to the foot. It seemed to glow as if the bones were made of red-hot metal. For over a month the foot had been quite painful, ever since I had hurt it in a minor traffic accident—a bone bruise, I assumed, and ignored it. But it had refused to go away. I decided to hypnotize myself and find out what the trouble was. I began with my usual self-hypnosis induction and, once in a trance, started asking myself questions using a technique called *ideomotor response:* If the answer to my question was yes, my right forefinger moved in response; if no, my left forefinger. Is my right foot healing? I asked, and my finger frantically signaled *NO!* Is there something wrong with my foot other than a bruise? I wondered. *YES,* came the immediate answer. Is it serious enough that I should see a doctor? *YES,* cried my body to myself. After I got out of the tank I made an appointment to see a foot doctor, who took an X-ray that showed a complete fracture of a major bone.

Self-hypnosis is easy. I picked it up in about a half hour from a popular paperback on the subject, and I have never demonstrated any talent at all for "psychic" activities. Generally when you speak of hypnosis, people visualize a wild-eyed Svengali imposing his twisted will on some gentle Trilby, or a poor fool, manipulated by a stage hypnotist, barking like a dog and running around on all fours. People imagine a deep and unconscious sleep, a surrender of self-control. At bottom, they think it's *weird*. Also, many look on self-hypnosis as some kind of mental feat akin to multiplying ten-digit numbers in your head: interesting, yes, but somehow suspect.

The truth is, hypnosis is a common mental state, one that most of us drift into and out of without even being aware of it, as we watch TV, read, listen to music, brush our teeth, drive our cars, ride on the subway, sunbathe, jog, or sit at our desks tapping our fingers. Not only is the hypnotic state normal, but it's very simple to enter. The two essential elements are *relaxation* and *focused attention*. Any time you have these two elements—whether you are shaving, spaced out on a TV commercial, or listening to a Beethoven piano concerto—you are likely to be in at least a mild hypnotic state. To make conscious use of the hypnotic state one more element is required: *suggestion*. Such as when that TV commercial shows stalwart moose hunters cracking open a frosty beer and you find yourself heaving up out of your easy chair and moseying robot-like to the refrigerator.

Hypersuggestibility. These are just examples of ordinary trance states and suggestions that go on without our awareness much of the time. But experiments have conclusively demonstrated that when someone becomes deeply relaxed—more so than is usual in day-to-day life and eliminates distractions by focusing attention on something, such as an object, a repeated word, music, then that person enters a state known as *hypersuggestibility* and whatever statements or suggestions are made to him enter directly into his mind, bypassing the mental filters and other mechanisms by which we usually judge such statements. The mind accepts suggestions, and virtually any information, so readily and completely when it is in a hypersuggestible state that many educators are capitalizing on the phenomenon by inducing the state in their students and then cramming astonishing amounts of information into their brains. Some language students, for example, are said to have learned, with total recall, thousands of new words in a single session. This technique, known as *superlearning*, is particularly useful for floaters.

There are a number of theories as to why the mind is so open in a hypersuggestible state. Some scientists trace it to the reticular activating system, which directs our attention and regulates our level of arousal. They suggest that when we are in a state of deep relaxation, with external stimuli eliminated or restricted by a focusing of attention, the RAS "turns up the volume" in certain receptive parts of the brain, so that when suggestions are made they are received directly and with greater volume (i.e., more attention and imputed value) than ordinarily.

Another theory, proposed by biofeedback expert Thomas Budzynski, traces hypersuggestibility to the difference in function between the left and right brains: In the relaxed state, with external awareness turned off, the usually dominant left hemisphere (in which much of our logical thought and word processing goes on) is restrained, while the right brain, seat of emotions and imagery, gains power, reaching a state of equilibrium with the left brain.

Thus, in the hypersuggestible state, the two hemispheres are working together, each half potentiating the other, so that the words of the suggestion are received and linked with deep emotional associations, the rational meaning of the words strengthened by the images they call forth from the right lobe. "Get access to the right hemispheres of individuals very quickly," says Budzynski, "and keep them in that state, and that's where a *lot of work gets done very quickly*. We get at this same place with float techniques, 'twilight learning,' subliminal processing, hypnosis, all of these."

Budzynski emphasizes that when the mind is in this relaxed state, with the dominance of the left hemisphere suspended and the right hemisphere functioning freely, it "has these properties of *uncritical acceptance of verbal material, or almost any material it can process*. What if you could cause a person to sustain that state, and not fall asleep? I believe floatation tanks are an ideal medium for doing that." [38]

People in hypnotic trance respond to suggestions in ways that seem hardly possible: When told they are becoming numb, they will experience total anesthesia; when told something hot is being touched to their skin, they will form immediate blisters. But in the floatation tank, everything is intensified. The relaxation is far deeper than any available outside the tank; the ability to concentrate is enormously enhanced, since there are no distractions; and as a result, receptivity to suggestions is increased dramatically.

Hypnosis expert and rest researcher Ian Wickramsekera, of the Eastern Virginia Medical School, delivered a paper at the First International Conference on REST and Self-Regulation, "Sensory Restriction and Self-Hypnosis as Potentiators of Self-Regulation," which presented evidence that sensory deprivation not only increases the depth of self-hypnosis, making the experience "much more vivid and more personally meaningful," but also results in more profound hypnotic effects, such as time distortion. The most significant discovery Wickramsekera made was that the chamber is very effective in helping people enter the hypnotic state who are not ordinarily receptive to, or able to enter, hypnosis. [260] This is supported by a study done by Arreed Barabasz, of Harvard Medical School, who used an isolation chamber to study hypnotic susceptibility, and concluded that "hypnotizability can be significantly and meaningfully enhanced by REST. Indeed, some [subjects] who initially scored in the lower ranges became hypnotic virtuosos ... ." When we consider that hypnotic suggestion can be used for a whole range of remarkable effects—such as helping people eliminate chronic pain, overcome illness, or undergo surgery without anesthesia and its accompanying dangers—the enhancement of hypnotizability caused by floating can be seen to have great significance. Barabasz touched on this in his conclusion: "Perhaps of more importance is the finding that the enhancement effect was significant and meaningful in its generalizability from the posthypnotic suggestion to greatly increased pain tolerance scores." [13]

Scripts, Programs, Habits.   Those who are wary of hypnotism should remember that we are all slipping in and out of light hypnotic trances all the time, and that our beliefs, self-images, in fact all our ideological baggage, are largely the result of hypnosis. If we see ourselves as sexually irresistible, threatened by the Russians, unlucky, or cursed with a violent temper, it's largely because we've been programmed, or hypnotized, to do so, through suggestions that have lodged themselves in our psyches in moments when we were particularly receptive or suggestible. Many of these suggestions, or "scripts," are a result of childhood experiences. Budzynski points out: "If you slap a child, or in any way get it into an altered state (and an altered state by definition seems to be more of a right hemisphere dominant state), and then say something to the child, you're going to be laying down a *script* in the right hemisphere, which may not have access later on to consciousness in the left hemisphere, but nevertheless will alter the behavior and attitudes of that child as an adult." Budzynski mentioned such scripts as "You're no good" and "You'll never amount to anything" as particularly powerful suggestions, leading to constant self-sabotage in adult life.[38] The question is not so much *whether* you want to be hypnotized as it is how conscious you are going to be of your hypnosis and how much control you will have over the suggestions or programs that enter your mind.

The difficulty in attempting to eliminate harmful programs, or decondition ourselves, is that our habits and beliefs tend to cling to us like leeches while we remain engaged in living our lives. It's difficult, for example, to decondition someone's habitual low self-esteem while he or she continues to circulate among people who seem to verify the negative self—perception. The answer, clearly, is to do the deconditioning while completely separated from the world in which one's habits and beliefs have their being. The most effective means of "getting away from it all" yet discovered is the float tank. It is the perfect deconditioning tool, since while we are floating we are completely separated from our normal relationship with the world, including our habitual responses, our conditioned acts and attitudes. And while deconditioning ourselves from the hypnotic baggage we've brought with us, we find that the tank is just as ideal for *recondition-*

ing—that is, hypnotizing ourselves and offering ourselves suggestions that counteract and supersede the unwanted beliefs and habits.

Even people convinced of the positive value of self-hypnosis often say regretfully, "Oh, but I could never do it," so certain are they that hypnosis requires some rare talent or knack. Hypnosis has been carefully and extensively observed and documented in experimental and clinical settings by scientists for over a century, and their conclusion is that under the proper conditions virtually *everyone* can be hypnotized. Psychoanalyst and hypnotherapist Dr. Roger Bernhardt writes, "anyone who is not neurologically impaired, retarded or psychotic can benefit from Self-hypnosis."[26] All that is required, Bernhardt insists, is a sincere desire to be hypnotized.

The reason many people feel themselves incapable of self-hypnosis is that successful self-hypnosis requires deep relaxation and the ability to concentrate so intently that external stimuli are ignored. Very few people other than those specially trained in meditation, progressive relaxation, and other mind/body control techniques, are able to fulfill these requirements, but the float tank provides them effortlessly. And as the studies of Wickramsekera and Barabasz show, floating is particularly successful in inducing a hypnotic state in people who are highly resistant to hypnosis outside the tank.

Induction. Outside the tank, the hypnotic induction process can be lengthy, but much of the time is spent in becoming progressively more deeply relaxed. In the tank, we can assume that by the time you want to induce hypnosis, you are already relaxed, either by letting go or by using one of the techniques described in the last chapter. Once you are relaxed, focus your attention on the process of hypnosis. There are countless ways of doing this, but these are among the most effective:

Counting Backward. Many hypnotists advise you to count backward from 100, but this is to ensure deep relaxation. In the tank you are already deeply relaxed and a shorter count works just as well, say from 10 down to zero. Count backward one number with each outbreath, and intersperse your counts with suggestions of increasing relaxation, increasing concentration, increasing suggestibility, and the repeated suggestion that when you reach zero you will be in a state of deep hypnosis.

Visualization of Sinking. My favorite induction method is one that takes me back to favorite diving spots on the barrier reefs of Belize and Central America. I visualize myself floating slowly downward through the clear

Caribbean waters. As I sink deeper and deeper, I look upward and watch the bottom of the boat grow smaller and smaller. I can see my air bubbles streaming slowly upward toward the surface after each breath. As I sink deeper I feel the water pressure increasing on my body. I seem to grow heavier. From the corners of my eyes I see coral cliffs, coming from below and then rising above me as I sink past the multicolored outcroppings. With each counted breath I sink deeper, suggesting to myself that I am becoming deeply hypnotized, and as I reach the bottom of the sea, several hundred feet down, I sink through an opening and continue deeper and deeper into the hole, watching my boat on the surface shrink to a speck....

Signal.   Most people find it helpful to have a hypnotic signal or *cue*, a special *trigger word* you use to indicate to yourself that you are *now*, at this instant, in hypnosis. Some like words with amusing connotations: *Shazam*, say, or *abracadabra*. Another favorite is *zero*—the logical end of your count, enabling you to give yourself repeated suggestions as you count down, such as "As I reach zero, I will be in a deep hypnotic trance." Whatever signal word you select, it lets you know that at that moment you are hypnotized, and you can then move on to making use of the hypnotic trance.

Suggestions.   Research shows that the hypnotic state is beneficial in itself, but in this it is little different from meditation or other kinds of deep relaxation. What distinguishes hypnosis from these other practices is its power to change behavior through suggestion. Suggestion lies at the root of all the astonishing powers of hypnosis, including total or local anesthesia, rapid self-healing, access to memories, body changes (such as disappearance of warts or tumors, or increased breast size), time distortion (making a few minutes seem like hours, or vice versa), age regression, strengthening the immune system, elimination of unwanted habits, elimination (or deconditioning, or deprogramming) of harmful attitudes such as lack of assertiveness, shyness, phobias, etc., and creation or strengthening of positive or desired attitudes and beliefs. Here are a few general principles that will enhance the effectiveness of suggestion in whatever context you wish to use it.

≈   *Repeat.* We all know the power of repetition from experience with insidious TV or radio commercials. By repeating your suggestion several times, perhaps using various wordings and images, you will increase its effectiveness.

≈ *Use present tense.* The unconscious mind appears to be very literal in interpreting our suggestions, so if you suggest that something *will* happen, your deepest conscious interprets this to mean that it is something in the future, i.e., *not now.* And the future, of course, is *always* not now. To suggest I *will recover from this illness* is to put recovery off until some indefinite tomorrow, while the suggestion *I am now in perfect health* or *I am now growing stronger and healthier* affirms that the process is already underway.

≈ *Suspend disbelief.* When you make suggestions, try to feel that they are, at least for the time being, completely true. Suppose you are suggesting you have great confidence at public speaking, when in fact it terrifies you. Try to experience your suggestions of confidence as absolutely true; create a mental image of yourself speaking with great poise and assurance; allow the physical experience to become real. Once you have experienced it as real in your imagination, your subconscious accepts it as real.

≈ *Be positive.* Positive suggestions have more force than negative ones, perhaps because the mere statement of the negative gives it substance. *I don't feel any desire to smoke* reminds us subconsciously that we do in fact have a desperate desire for a cigarette, while *I feel so energetic and clearheaded when I am not smoking* emphasizes the positive, creating a mental image in which smoking itself is not present. Research into the differing capabilities of the two hemispheres of the brain shows that the visual-oriented right hemisphere is able to comprehend spoken language but does not process negatives very well. So, if we're trying to bypass the logical brain and get into the deeper and more unconscious levels of the mind, we must speak in a language that every part of the brain can understand.

≈ *Be concrete and specific.* Rather than making suggestions about general attitudes—*I am full of confidence*, or *I am successful in whatever I do*—deal with specific circumstances, seeing yourself confidently performing that recital, giving that speech, successfully making a certain sale, or passing a required test. Brain researchers have discovered that, in the words of Thomas Budzynski, "Right hemisphere speech comprehension is simple, concrete, nothing abstract—it doesn't seem to process abstract material at all." [38]

≈ *Visualize.* Suggestions are much more potent when linked with an appropriate visual image. *See* the boffo review of your performance in the local newspaper. *See* the healing energy pouring into that broken ankle. *See* yourself capably handling that business negotiation. This ensures that your suggestion is implanted firmly in the visually oriented right hemisphere as well as in the verbal left, so that the suggestion is imbued with emotional energy and engages your entire mind. Also, there is evidence that any visual image held in your mind firmly enough is accepted into your permanent memory as if it were a real experience; remember the experiments in which boys who visualized themselves shooting basketballs improved as much as those who actually practiced free throws every day.

≈   *Find the rhythm.* There is now evidence that suggestions are more effective when they are stated rhythmically, and linked to your own rhythms. Repeat your suggestions in a kind of internal poetry or song, in phrases that come easily, repeated in a way that harmonizes with your breathing. Brain researchers have found that voice intonation and rhythm are processed by the right hemisphere. People who are largely left-brain oriented often talk in a monotonous, unrhythmic way, while those who are skilled in gaining access to the right hemisphere—like gospel preachers—speak with powerful rhythms and great variation in voice intonation. (Compare, for example, the speech patterns of Henry Kissinger and Martin Luther King, Jr.) The rhythm and intonation of suggestions is particularly important to those who are preparing tapes of suggestions to listen to while in the tank.

Measuring Depth of Hypnosis.   One frequent question is, "How do you know when you're hypnotized?" The answer is that generally you just know: The deeply relaxed state of calm, alert lucidity and control is recognizable. With practice it becomes very familiar. However, there are a number of tests that have the added value of deepening your trance at the same time they verify it. Among them are:

≈   *Eye closure.* Simply suggest to yourself that your eyelids are firmly shut, that the lids are sealed, that no matter how hard you might try to open your eyelids they will remain closed—in fact, the harder you try to open your eyelids the more tightly they will remain closed. Repeat this suggestion over and over in various forms and wordings, adding visual images (perhaps a golden needle stitching the lids shut with silver thread, or glue oozing out of a tube onto your eyelids and sealing them shut). Finally, suggest that at a given signal you will *try* to open your eyelids (the word *try* is important, since it implies failure) but will not be able to. Add to this the suggestion that when you try to open your eyelids and are unable to, it will be a signal for you to fall even deeper into hypnosis. When you try to open your lids you will find that the muscles seem paralyzed. Accept this and feel yourself falling even deeper into hypnosis.

≈   *Ideomotor response.* This is the method I used to interrogate myself about my ankle. Ask yourself questions, and answer with predetermined body movements, such as moving the right forefinger to mean yes, left fore-finger for no, right thumb, "I don't want to answer the question"; left thumb, "I don't know." Some of the answers you get will astonish you, but it doesn't mean your body is inhabited by an alien spirit. It is simply your subconscious or unconscious mind directing the movements of your body to convey infor-mation that you are not consciously aware of: a sort of hypnotic Ouija board.

Ultimately, the whole question of depth is of little importance. Hypnotists stress that level of trance does not significantly affect the power of your suggestions: Even in a light trance suggestions work very well. Suggestions made just in a state of deep relaxation are still quite effective and long-lasting. Concern about whether you're actually hypnotized, and if so how deep your trance is, can be counterproductive. The best approach is the same one used for floating in general: Simply let go of striving, and allow yourself to sink as deep as you can without effort.

Implant a Cue Word. After you have given yourself the appropriate sugges-tions for changing behavior, and before you are ready to emerge from the trance state, implant a suggestion that will help you return easily to a trance at any time you wish by using your personal trance signal word. Pay attention to how you feel—relaxed, focused, alert and suggest that you will be able to hypnotize yourself and return to this state at any time you wish, simply by saying your trance induction word. Suggest that each time you hypnotize yourself you become more skilled and proficient at self-hypnosis; each time you go to a deeper level of trance more easily and rapidly than before.

Emerging from Trance. There is usually no pressing need to emerge from the trance while floating. When you have finished your hypnotic suggestions, simply relax, with the thought that when your float session is over you will emerge from the tank alert, relaxed, clearheaded, peaceful, and feeling won-derful. At no time is there any chance you will go into a trance and not come out. This is impossible, since you are quite conscious at all times, and should there be any need for you to act quickly, you will immediately emerge from the trance clearheaded and ready to act effectively and rationally.

EIGHTEEN

FLOATING FOR RELIEF OF PAIN

Jan is a vibrant young filmmaker. When I first spoke to her she was so happy and healthy I would have bet she'd never known a sick day in her life. However, Jan suffers from rheumatoid arthritis. When her boyfriend had given her a surprise present of a float session she had gone for her first float with some fear. While she was in the tank an unexpected thing happened: She felt the familiar arthritis pain in her lower back turn into a bright, intensely glowing ball of light. Jan focused on the shimmering spot and felt the pain disappear. "It was about forty minutes into the float, and then, well, time just disappeared—you know, there was just no sense of time at all until they were knocking on the tank and telling me my hour was up." It wasn't until a few days later that she remembered the glowing ball of light in her back, and realized she had been free of pain since getting out of the tank. When I spoke with her several weeks later she had floated three times and was eager to begin doing floats longer than an hour.

"When I broke several bones in a bicycle accident," recalled John C. Lilly, the developer and first explorer of the floatation tank, "I went for five days without sleep before finally resorting to the tank in desperation. There, I was free from the pain, without drugs, for the first time since I had the accident. That's because a tank frees up all the pain due to gravity." [86]

In Phoenix, Arizona, seventeen former manual laborers who had suffered disabling injuries that were intractable to surgery, many of them victims of chronic pain, were put through a sixty-hour therapy course that centered on immersion in floatation tanks. After the floating regimen, fourteen of them were able to return to work—many for the first time in years—with remission of pain, and recoveries the men's employer called "on the order of miraculous." Psychophysiologist Harold Cairn, Ph.D., of Wellness Research Associates, claims that a follow-up after two years confirms the remission.[41]

I could continue with scores of stories like these, since almost everyone I spoke with about floating had his or her own favorite "how floating cured my headache" story. No one, including scientists who have done tank research, seems to have any doubts that floatation has remarkable and long-lasting analgesic effects. The question is, why?

The Admirable Endorphins

I first put that question to Gary Higgins, the president of Float to Relax, Incorporated, a company that manufactures and sells floatation tanks and has opened commercial float centers all across the United States, and which at that time operated a laboratory engaged in researching the effects of floatation on such things as blood chemistry, brain waves, and muscular tension. "We believe a chemical change occurs in the body when relaxation is reached," said Higgins. "People do receive relief from chronic pain, and we believe the reason they do is that relaxation stimulates the production of the body's own opiates, or pain-killers. We're now involved in research to study the long-term benefits of the increased production of these pain-killers, beta endorphins, and we associate it with relief from migraine headaches, low back pain, sports-related injuries, arthritis, and so on."

I'd heard about these admirable endorphins. Research indicated that a runner's brain pours a sizable dollop of the pain-killers into the system after about thirty or forty minutes of running, and that they are probably the cause of the well-known "runner's high." I decided to investigate this remarkable biochemical, which seems to be literally the "opiate of the people." The story, I found, unreeled like a cracking good whodunit, complete with deucedly singular puzzles and unsolved mysteries.

First, it's important to understand how messages travel through the unthinkably complex network of the brain's nerve cells. Scientists now estimate that the brain contains some 100 billion of these cells, called *neurons*—about the number of stars in the galaxy. Most importantly, no two of these neurons are exactly alike. Each neuron has a central core or body from which sprout numerous long wispy filaments known as *dendrites*, which form bushy trees with intricately interlaced branches around the cell body. Also extending from the cell body is a single stringy fiber, the *axon*, which branches into numerous filaments. Dendrites receive incoming signals and carry them to the cell body; the cell body emits outgoing signals, and the axon carries the signals to the numerous axon terminals, where the signals are passed on to many dendrites of many other neurons.

A single neuron receives signals from hundreds or thousands of other neurons, and it sends messages on to hundreds or thousands of other neurons. Each neuron is as complex as an entire small computer. From each of these billions of computers, information received from thousands of other computers is passed on to thousands of other computers, which are in turn connected to thousands of other neurons, making in all as many as one quadrillion connections, forming an interwoven fabric of such incomprehensible richness and complexity that the human brain has a larger number of potential connections among its cells (i.e., a larger number of potential mental states) than the total number of atomic particles in the universe.

With each unique cell sending several impulses per second, the brain is continually humming with billions of impulses—truly, in the words of one brain scientist, an "enchanted loom," the vastest, most intricate, and ultimately most mysterious communications network that has ever existed.

The impulses by which neurons communicate are carried from the cell body down the axon to the numerous axon terminals, or buttons, by means of electrical impulses. But there is a microscopic gap between the tip of each axon terminal and the receptor region on the dendrite of the cell next in line. This gap is known as a *synapse*, and for messages to be transmitted across the gap the electrical impulses must be translated into chemicals. When a sufficient electrical impulse reaches the end of one nerve, that nerve end is stimulated to release a complex neurochemical, a long and uniquely twisted and sequenced pattern of amino acids. This neurochemical crosses the gap to the receiving dendrite of another neuron, where there are complex strings of amino acids called *receptor sites*. These receptors are shaped and twisted into a specific pattern, with amino acids arranged in such a way that only their perfect complement will "fit," or bind itself to the site. It's because the neurochemicals must have the identical amino acid pattern as the receptors to become attached, that the process has been compared to fitting a key into a lock.

Once the proper molecule has fit into the receptor, the lock is opened; the receptor is stimulated into action: A message is transmitted from one cell to the next. The chemicals that carry these messages across the synapses are known as *neurotransmitters*. And while scientists have discovered just over fifty neurotransmitters since 1975, they now believe there must be many more, each one having an important role in influencing our moods and feelings, carrying messages for us to feel happy, to suffer pain, to remember, to be depressed.

The Keys of Paradise.　So, to return to our story, imagine their surprise when, in 1973, scientists made the amazing discovery that our brain cells contain receptor sites specifically designed to receive opiates. Heroin, morphine, opium, methadone, Demerol, and other such drugs fit right into these *opiate receptors*, like keys fitting perfectly into matching locks.

But here was a real mystery: The brain evolved millions of years ago (the opiates affect other vertebrates as they do humans, so we know that the receptor sites evolved many millions of years back), so how could it have these complex receptor sites that seem specifically suited for opiate drugs, which have only been in use some few thousands of years? What on earth are we doing with specially designed drug sites wired into our brains? They say that if God had wanted us to fly He would have given us wings; well, here was proof that He had given us drug receptors. Surely He didn't intend for us to become junkies. The scientists decided that the existence of opiate receptors meant that the brain must produce its own version of these drugs—natural painkillers, our own chemical key to fit our receptor lock, secreted by the brain's neurons. Such a key, able to unlock the secrets of pain, pleasure, addiction, and mental illness, would surely be something very like the key to paradise. The search was on.

In 1975 scientists discovered *enkephalins* (from the Greek for "in the head"), each enkephalin a string of intricately structured amino acids that fit the opiate receptors perfectly and have opiate-like effects. It was soon discovered that each enkephalin was just a part of a much longer and more complex molecule. Part of this long molecule had even more powerful analgesic effects and was more long-lasting in the body than enkephalins. This molecule was called *beta endorphin*, from the words *endogenous morphine* (that is, morphine produced internally). In the years since 1975, others of these natural opiates have been discovered. Produced by the brain, beta endorphin, and others of these natural drugs, seem to be released in situations of comfort as well as pain, are many times more powerful than morphine, and remain active in the body for hours.

This was big news. For over a century scientists had been searching for specific links between brain biochemistry and human behavior, and with the discovery of the endorphins the link was established. In the words of Candace Pert, one of the discoverers of the opiate receptors, now at the National Institutes of Mental Health: "There used to be two systems of knowledge: hard science—chemistry, physics, biophysics—on the one hand, and, on the other, a system of knowledge that included ethology, psychology, and psychiatry. And now it's as if a lightning bolt had connected the two. It's all one system—neuroscience." [102] Or, as her NIMH colleague Michael Brownstein put it: "This is a fun time to be doing neuroscience. A lot of good people see it as the last frontier." [104]

In the few years since the discovery of the endorphins, scientists have found they serve an astonishing variety of functions, including relieving pain, causing pleasure, and filtering, selecting, and integrating information input from the senses. To return to the question of God's inscrutable purposes in giving us opiate receptors, doctor and essayist Lewis Thomas ponders why the "enthralling" endorphins exist at all, not only in humans but in all vertebrates, even in worms:

> Yet there it is, a biologically universal act of mercy. I cannot explain it, except to say that I would have put it in had I been around at the very beginning, sitting as a member of a planning committee, say, and charged with the responsibility for organizing for the future a closed ecosystem crowded with an infinite variety of life on this planet. No such system could possibly operate without pain, and pain receptors would have to be planned in detail for all sentient forms of life, plainly for their own protection and the avoidance of danger. But not limitless pain; this would have the effect of turbulence, unhinging the whole system in an agony even before it got underway.... I would have cast a vote for a modulator of pain.... In this sense, endorphin may have developed in our brains not for its selective value to our species, or any species, or any individuals without species, but for the survival and perpetuation of the whole biosphere, or as it is sometimes called, the System.[250]

Endorphins offered explanations for many occurrences which had baffled scientists. For example, acupuncture—inserting needles into specific parts of the body and manipulating them in certain ways. In both laboratory and clinical settings it had been conclusively shown that acupuncture blocked pain; the Chinese had been using it for thousands of years, but no one could explain how it worked. Then researchers decided to see how the drug *naloxone* affected the pain-killing abilities of acupuncture. Naloxone is a drug that has a structure virtually identical to the opiates, and fits right into the opiate receptors of the brain, but it has none of the pain-killing or pleasant effects of the opiates. By binding to the opiate receptors, naloxone fills up all the available receptors and blocks the entry of the real opiates, thus keeping any opiates in the system from having any effects. Since it keeps the opiate "message" from getting through, naloxone is known as an *opiate antagonist*. Since the endorphins are opiates, their effects are blocked by naloxone. When people who had been anesthetized by acupuncture were administered naloxone, acupuncture no longer deadened their pain. The conclusion: Acupuncture gets its anesthetic power by somehow stimulating the brain to secrete endorphins.[1,137,163]

Many who have studied acupuncture believe it works through influencing the body's electrical systems. One of the most exciting new developments in neuroscience and medicine has been *electrotherapy:* Many doctors and medical researchers have treated sufferers of chronic, intractable pain by electrically stimulating parts of their brains. Doctors have found that just a few minutes of stimulation of certain brain areas can provide pain relief lasting twelve hours or more. Exactly how this electrical analgesia worked was a mystery. Again the opiate antagonist naloxone was administered, and suddenly electrical stimulation no longer alleviated the pain. The conclusion: The way electricity turns off pain is by stimulating the brain to produce a flood of endorphins.[193] (Later tests analyzing body fluids confirmed this, showing endorphin levels increased eightfold after electrical stimulation.)

Electrical stimulation of the brain brings up a classic series of experiments carried out in the 1950s by Dr. James Olds, who discovered a certain area in the hypothalamus of a white rat that, when electrically stimulated, seemed to cause the rat intense pleasure. Ingeniously, Olds wired up the rats so they could stimulate their own pleasure centers by pressing a foot pedal. The rats immediately began an orgy of self-stimulation, pressing the pedals as often as five thousand times an hour, and gladly underwent all sorts of horrible experiences for the chance to press the pleasure pedal.[174, 175] The scientists were intrigued. What in the world could be so very, very pleasurable?

With the discovery of the endorphins, and the experiments that followed which showed how electrical stimulation of the brain produced a release of endorphins, the answer has become more clear. Many neuroscientists now suggest that the natural opiates are "the brain's own internal reward system."[102] The rats were engaged in an activity that caused the release of pleasure in their brains, and, in the words of neuroscientist Candace Pert: "When humans engage in various activities, neurojuices associated either with pleasure or with pain are released." And as the well-known pleasures of opiates cause humans to behave like electrically wired white rats, so our internal opiates, whether stimulated electrically or by whirling acupuncture needles, are apparently not just analgesic but also powerfully euphoric.

The Reign of Pain Stays Mainly in the Brain. The increased levels of endorphins and enkephalins we have discussed thus far have been in some way externally stimulated. However, we now know that humans are also capable of releasing large quantities of endorphins into their systems simply by assuming a certain state of mind.

One of the most amazing—and baffling—medical phenomena has been the ability of humans to alleviate pain and heal themselves of virtually any illness merely by taking a medication or treatment which they believe to be beneficial, but which (unbeknownst to them) has no intrinsic therapeutic value—such as a sugar pill. This mysterious curative factor, rooted somehow in the power of suggestion, is known as the *placebo effect*.

The sicknesses and pain the people suffered were not "in their heads" or imaginary; they were very real and often serious, and the placebo effect mobilized quite real and powerful physiological forces in their bodies. Just what those forces were, however, was a mystery. Now a part of that mystery has been solved; a number of studies have clearly demonstrated that the pain relief of the placebo effect is a product of increased levels of endorphins, released by the body in response to the placebo.

In one study, patients were given two injections of "pain-killers" after oral surgery, with the injections several hours apart. The injections were either morphine, naloxone, or a placebo. Of particular interest were the subjects who responded to the placebo. It eliminated their pain as effectively as morphine; however, when they were given their second shot—this time of naloxone — they immediately felt significantly more pain. The obvious conclusion, then, is that the placebo worked by causing the people who received it to release internal opiates. Other experiments have confirmed this conclusion.[1,137,163]

When results like these began to be widely known, in the mid and late 1970s, people began to understand the incredible implications: The human mind, "thoughts," had the power to trigger endorphin release. Said Kenneth Pelletier:

> It is becoming increasingly clear that psychological processes produce detectable variations in the electrical and biochemical activity of the entire central nervous system. Minute electromagnetic potentials appear to govern basic biological functions manifested in recovery from injury as well as regenerations. Biological processes can be influenced directly by manipulation of these electrical potentials through electrical stimulation and classic acupuncture. Perhaps the perineural DC system is the link between human consciousness and its influence on the endorphin and enkephalin response as manifested in the placebo response as well as certain aspects of spontaneous remission.

Understanding of this link may make it possible systematically to direct consciousness to regulate these internal electrical and biochemical processes, in a manner analogous to the now common practices of clinical biofeedback.[188]

In the words of another scientist: "Perhaps the most intriguing question is whether this system can be activated voluntarily; that is, can people will themselves to feel less pain or learn some mental trick to set the pain-suppressing mechanism in motion?" [72]

And, knowing the intensity of pleasure these internal opiates can bring in addition to their analgesic effects, we can add this intriguing question: "Can this pleasure system be activated voluntarily; that is, can people will themselves to feel intense pleasure or learn some mental trick to set the pleasure-bringing mechanism in motion?"

We now know that the answer to these questions is yes: We can voluntarily set our pain-relief and pleasure mechanisms in motion—that is, we can learn mental tricks, and will ourselves to release endorphins, as well as other beneficial neurochemicals. And the most effective tool yet found for accomplishing these ends is the floatation tank.

Floating Out Endorphins

Let's return to Gary Higgins's assertion that one explanation for the pain-relief effects of the tank is that the state of deep relaxation you attain while floating causes the body to release endorphins. Is this true? I wondered. For if it is, it would explain not only the analgesic effects of floatation but also the strong flood of pleasure many floaters describe; and it would touch as well on all those other areas in which endorphins seem to have a powerful influence, such as enabling those addicted to certain drugs or behaviors to break their addictions, heightening learning capacity, deflecting painful psychological experiences, enhancing orgasm, and much more.

In fact, endorphin researcher Candace Pert, in a talk with writer Judith Hooper, says that endorphins actually determine what "reality" is for each of us, and how much of it to let in: "Our team at NIMH," she says, "has proposed that the endorphins, our natural opiates, are a filtering mechanism in the brain. The opiate system selectively filters incoming information from every sense—sight, hearing, smell, taste, and touch—and blocks some of it from percolating up to higher levels of consciousness. Nobody really knows what the world looks like, as philosophers like Bishop Berkeley and David Hume observed. Everybody's version of the world is significantly different."

Intriguingly, it is in the limbic system that opiate receptors are most densely packed; and since the limbic brain operates in terms of emotions, this leads Pert to believe that endorphins "filter incoming information and place it in an emotional context. We evaluate environmental signals according to the limbic standards of pleasure and pain.... Through the endorphin system you decide what aspects of reality to pay attention to. And the criteria for deciding aren't ones that you and I made up last week—they're criteria that our ancestors worked out about a million years ago.

"The stimuli your brain selects as important are those that will have the most survival value, not just for you but for your children.... All these little decisions have to be tied into the limbic system, tied in to sex and violence— whom to make love to and whom to kill." Citing differences in behavior between the sexes, Pert contends that these are in part the result of endorphins: men and women derive pleasure from, and the endorphins of the ancient, limbic or visceral brain cause them to pay attention to, different aspects of reality. And while the largest numbers of endorphins and opiate receptors are found in the limbic brain, we have seen that it is exactly in the limbic brain that floating seems to have its most powerful influence.[102]

The wide range of effects of endorphins seems so similar to the effects of floatation—pain relief, pleasure, a discernible alteration in the "reality" being experienced, a keen sense of being in touch with deeper, older drives, emotions, and levels of the mind—that purely on anecdotal grounds one suspects there must be a link. But anecdotes do not constitute proof. Is there any solid scientific evidence linking floating with increases in endorphins? I raised the question in a conversation with Thomas Fine, of the department of Psychiatry at the Medical College of Ohio. Fine has established a REST laboratory and Behavioral Medicine Clinic at MCO where he uses floatation tanks for clinical treatment and has done extensive laboratory research on the effects of floatation, in conjunction with neuroendocrinologist John Turner. When I asked about endorphins, Fine told me about an experiment he and Turner had recently conducted.

He and three other researchers—all experienced floaters—had each taken a series of four floating sessions in the clinic's tanks. Before each float, the floater was given an injection. Each injection was either a placebo or naloxone, administered in double-blind protocol, so that neither the floater nor the person who administered the injection knew what it contained. After each of the four floats, the floater was asked to guess whether he had been given naloxone or a placebo. A placebo, of course, would have no discernible effect on the float, while naloxone, as an opiate antagonist, would bind to the brain's opiate receptors and block any pain-killing or pleasure-causing effects that would result from the release of endorphins. Therefore, if floating did *not* release endorphins, there should be no way to tell the naloxone from the placebo. If floating does in fact cause the release of endorphins, experienced floaters would easily be able to tell the naloxone, since it would keep them from feeling the usual euphoric/analgesic effects. The four subjects guessed what they had been injected with after each of four floats, a total of sixteen guesses. The results: Sixteen out of sixteen "guesses" were correct!

"This is not conclusive," Fine cautioned me, emphasizing that the experiment had been a sort of preliminary test to see if there were grounds to conduct a full-blown experiment. Among the methodological weaknesses Fine mentioned was that floatation enhances sensory awareness, so that if there were any subtle side effects of naloxone, the floater would become more aware of them than a person ordinarily would (perhaps naloxone leads to the release of epinephrine and norepinephrine). So the 100 percent accuracy of the floaters' guesses could possibly come from their perception of the *presence* of naloxone, rather than from their awareness of the *lack* of endorphins. "But there was no doubt about it," Fine said. "You just knew when you had naloxone— I just didn't feel anything at all like I do when I usually float." He agreed that while the test was only "suggestive" and not conclusive, its implications were striking, even exciting.

Anxiety, Pleasure, and Pain

"The mind is its own place, and in itself can make a heaven of hell, and a hell of heaven." Research psychologists continue to demonstrate that Milton's perceptions are correct, whether we see the mind as merely some adjunct to the physical brain or as a separate phenomenon. We know now, for example, that our state of mind determines the "painfulness" of pain; that anxiety can increase the painfulness of a given stimulus while pleasure can decrease the painfulness of the same stimulus. In experiments by Harris Hill and colleagues at the U.S. Public Health Service Hospital in Lexington, Kentucky, subjects had their anxiety dispelled by reassurances that they were in control of a pain-producing stimulus (a steadily increasing level of electric shock or burning heat); it was found that the pain-producing stimulus was perceived as significantly less painful than the very same stimulus under conditions of high anxiety, in which the subjects did not have direct control over the stimulus and had to rely on the experimenter.

One of the most consistent effects of floatation is a dramatic decrease in anxiety, both as subjectively perceived by the floater and as measured against certain physiological scales of anxiety (including blood pressure; levels of ACTH, adrenaline, and noradrenaline; pulse; oxygen consumption; and galvanic skin response). Therefore, floatation's proven ability to decrease anxiety can significantly reduce the painfulness of life's everyday pain-producing stimuli, whether it is a headache, a broken bone, or a broken heart. It's beginning to look as if the specific remedy for any irruption of pain in your life is to find your way quickly to the nearest float tank, plop in, and spend an hour pumping up your endorphin levels and avoiding the pain-increasing effects of anxiety.

Putting the Reptile to Sleep. In our discussion of the triune brain theory, we noted that part of the earliest evolved reptile brain is the reticular activating system, which has the essential function of arousing the higher parts of the brain. In addition, the RAS has the further interesting function of controlling selective attention: It determines whether we will pay attention to internal or external stimulation, and anyone who has had the experience of forgetting about a painful injury while enthralled by a ripping good book or movie has firsthand experience of how the RAS can shift awareness. In regulating the flow of information to the brain, the RAS turns the pitch of our sensations up or down. These adjustments of sensory volume are often determined by the novelty or irrelevance of a particular sensation. At every moment, all over our bodies, our senses are being stimulated by our clothes pressing against us, yet the RAS decides that such information is irrelevant and screens it from our attention, while the almost weightless pressure of a mosquito on a single hair will be immediately noticed.

It should not be surprising, then, that the RAS also regulates pain sensation. In fact, of all our sensations, pain is the one most inextricably bound up with consciousness, awareness, arousal, and attention. We recognize this link in our language, when we speak of being "painfully aware." Other sensations do not necessarily demand our attention—we can have chronic pleasure or chronic touch or even chronic boredom and yet continue our normal lives, but chronic pain is somehow different. It seems to nag, to wheedle, to insist. Intense pain brings with it feelings of urgency and excitement, as the RAS rings its alarm bell to get our attention.

Since pain is so wrapped up with awareness, it follows naturally that when we do have pain and somehow succeed in turning our awareness to something else, the pain recedes or disappears; again the RAS has regulated the pain by deciding not to bring it to our attention. So it makes sense that, in the words of neurosurgeon George Ojemann of the University of Washington School of Medicine: "One way to control severe pain would be to change the reticular activating system so that it turns down the sensitivity in pain pathways."[42] But how does one go about getting the RAS to "turn down" pain?

The relation between floating and the RAS was drawn by Gregg Jacobs, Robert Heilbronner, and John Stanley, researchers at Lawrence University, in an experiment whose purpose was to find the effects of floatation on relaxation. Dividing twenty-eight subjects into two groups, the researchers put one group through ten forty-five-minute sessions in a floatation tank over a period of weeks, while the other group also had ten relaxation sessions but did not go into a floatation tank. Measurements of muscular tension and blood pressure were made before and after each session, with the subjects who used the floatation tank registering significant and "impressive" decreases in both. The researchers sought some explanation for the dramatic mind/body changes brought about by floating, and focused on the RAS. They concluded by suggesting that floating "decreases the activity level of the reticular activating system and, subsequently, the cortex and hypothalamus, which are integral to the stress reaction in response to external stimuli. This decrease in activation can foster a shift of attention toward an internal mode of consciousness conducive to meditation and relaxation."[111] Or as these researchers put it in another paper: "It would appear that a reduction in sensory input facilitates physiological relaxation by decreasing sensory input to the reticular activating system. Since the reticular activating system receives less input, it sends fewer arousing signals to the cortex, which, in turn, decreases neural firings to subcortical regions of the brain responsible for the flight or fight response, specifically the hypothalamus."[112]

One way of looking at this is to say that, just as the RAS switches our attention from external to internal stimuli—or from an outer-directed state to an inner-directed state—when it receives less input from our sensory apparatus (the body), as it does when we are floating, so also the RAS turns our attention away from the body, and whatever physical pain it might be suffering, toward an internal state in which we are not aware of the body.

This loss of body awareness is not simply a feeling of being more interested in your thoughts; at a certain point in the float there is a distinct and noticeable feeling of no longer having a body at all. It seems evident that this phenomenon is the result of the RAS firmly turning awareness away from the body, where nothing seems to be happening to the inner state. With this turning inward, all feeling of pain disappears.

No Time for Pain.   One of the fascinating characteristics of "tank time" is that it seems completely unrelated to "real world time." Most floaters find that the first few minutes of tank time seem quite normal, but then awareness of the passage of time becomes distorted. Certain streams of images or mental experiences can seem to take hours, and yet when you emerge from these states it seems in fact as if no time has passed.

This loss of time-awareness is a consistent characteristic of the theta state, and tests have shown that a floater in the deep relaxation of the tank generates large amounts of theta waves. It is interesting to consider the links between the ability to stop the flow of time when in the tank and the pain relief we get from floating. One person who has done extensive clinical research into the relationship between time and pain is Dr. Larry Dossey, chief of staff of Medical City Dallas Hospital. "Persons who experience pain," observes Dossey in his book *Space, Time & Medicine,* "ordinarily live in a contracted or constricted time sense. Minutes seem like hours when one is hurting. Because the time sense is constricted, pain is magnified—sometimes far beyond what seems appropriate."

This is a phenomenon we're all familiar with: Time flies when you're having fun. Dossey has done research with this plastic, stretchable nature of time, noting that virtually all the ways we use to control pain have something to do with manipulating our sense of time, including medications that make us "float" or feel "drowsy," as well as hypnosis, biofeedback, meditation, and progressive relaxation. In fact, he concludes, clinical experience shows that "*any* device or technique that expands one's sense of time can be used as an analgesic!"

By what mechanism does modifying time work to alleviate pain? Dossey suggests that the experience of time expansion and the analgesia are both results of "actual changes in brain physiology," including the release in the brain of endorphins.[62] Once again we see floating, consciousness, and biochemistry interacting to bring about an expansion in human powers.

This plasticity of time Dossey sees as so important — the sense of freedom from time, freedom within time—is also a distinguishing characteristic of "flow," the element Mihaly Csikszentmihalyi finds present in all activity that is intrinsically enjoyable: that state in which action and awareness merge, attention is centered on a limited stimulus field, and one experiences self-forgetfulness or loss of self-consciousness and becomes more intensely aware of internal processes.

There is an extraordinary linkage taking place here: Somehow, flow experience (which we have noted includes religious and transcendental experience, as well as play, fun, adventure, and exploration); "timeless" or "out of time" experience and the ability to modify or expand our perception of time at will; the ability to intentionally manipulate and eliminate pain; and the related ability to intentionally manipulate and intensify pleasure—all are a part of some central process whose nexus is regulation of the chemistry of the brain, particularly the release of endorphins and other bliss-producing substances. And what Dossey, Csikszentmihalyi, Pelletier, Pert, and others are saying is that this regulation of the chemistry of the brain is something that we can *learn to control*; that, consciously or unconsciously, through training or instinct, and whether we like it or not, we are all engaged in a constant process of self-regulation of our brain chemistry.

Whether we accomplish it by choosing our favorite flow experience (sport, hobby, game, religion), by manipulating time, or by engaging in some self-regulation activity like meditation or relaxation, we are all involved in regulating the flow of certain powerful and pleasurable chemicals in the brain. And what I am suggesting—what the evidence indicates—is that the floatation tank is the most direct, rapid, efficient, foolproof, effective way to regulate the flow of these chemicals.

Indications are that the body responds to floating by naturally increasing the level of endorphins in the body. Simply floating, without any conscious mind-control techniques, does reduce pain. However, using the techniques of visualization and suggestion described in earlier chapters, floaters should be able to learn consciously to increase the amount of endorphins released in the brain.

NINETEEN

IMPROVING ATHLETIC PERFORMANCE

Herbie had tried for several years to finish the New York Marathon in under three hours. But each year he would push too hard, his body would rebel, and Herbie would end up running with shin splints, stress fracture, inflamed knee, or whatever that year's injury was. He began to think that breaking what he called the three-hour barrier was simply beyond his capacity. Then last year he discovered the float tank. "It worked for me in a number of ways," Herbie says. "I'd go in the tank and watch myself running—I'd be dissociated, watching my body from above or from the side, like a videotape. I could observe myself objectively, see how I was holding my head, what my arm swing was like, and this helped me cut out a lot of wasted motion. Also, in the tank I became intensely aware of tensions or stresses in my body even before they became physically noticeable—I could tell when my hamstring was tight, so I could stretch that specific spot, and I could tell when I was pushing too hard, overtraining, so I could cut back a bit. As a result of this fine-tuning I had no injuries at all. A first for me.

"Also, every time I floated I'd visualize myself crossing the finish line up in Central Park—you know, the cheering multitudes, the TV cameras. I'd even smell the hot dogs and feel the cool air. And there I am, running strongly, crossing under the clock, and I can see the clock is 2:50, fifteen minutes better than my personal best. Also, whenever I'd feel tired, I'd come in for a float, and it seemed to help me get the spring back in my legs fast." Herbie made it to the marathon without injuries that year. His finishing time was about 2:50.

As the 1981 NFL season began, Dallas Cowboy placekicker Rafael Septien had an undiagnosed hernia that spread such pain and stiffness through his legs, abdomen, and back that Coach Tom Landry thought he might have to find a new kicker. However, the Cowboys had just acquired a float tank, and Rafael discovered that floating not only relaxed him and helped relieve the pain but also increased his ability to concentrate.

Kicking demands total concentration and confidence, and Rafael had begun reading books on positive thinking and visualization. He found that the tank increased his ability to visualize and the power of his positive suggestions. As he floated, he saw himself kicking perfect field goals, and repeated, "I am my own authority. I only let the most fine thoughts enter my mind and spirit. ... I have done it over and over. I *know* if I put my left foot in the right position and keep my head down and follow through I will kick all my field goals, or at least ninety percent of them."

Despite his injury, Septien opened the season with a string of perfect field goals, at one point had kicked twenty-two out of twenty-four, and capped a spectacular season by being selected All-Pro.

Since then, Septien has incorporated audio- and videotapes into his float. The audio tapes play relaxation and positive thinking messages; the videotapes show him kicking perfect field goals, and are played over and over through a video monitor attached to the top of the tank. He believes his daily floats are the key to his success: "No doubt about it," he told me. "If you conquer doubt and fear, you conquer failure. If you don't doubt, if you know you're going to do it, it's easier. Your muscles are more relaxed, and then you perform what you have practiced in the tank."

Neurophysiologist Dr. Jeffrey Gmelch, of Columbia University, has reasons to be both personally and professionally interested in sports medicine and the effects of floating. His practice involves much work in physical rehabilitation of stroke victims and other disabled people, and he is a dedicated runner. "I'm not a competitive runner," he told me, "but I did find that I could run much more easily for a week or two after floating. I tend to look at things as a scientist, so seen physiologically it's because of the buildup of lactic acid—it's lactic acid that causes fatigue and muscle soreness, and after those two weeks the lactic acid builds up and the effects of the float tend to wear off. I'm sure it's also that the body is relaxed after you get out for a number of days or even weeks after that you still feel the effects of it. It's a long-term alteration in the metabolism.

"So I *did* notice better athletic performance from the tank. It improved my ease in movement, even just walking around. I normally have stress in my upper back, especially if I run. And for a week or two after I float, I don't experience it. For a time there I was floating every two weeks, and during that period I felt no strain or tension in running. I generally get a cramp in my right shoulder and upper back which will make me stop running or cut my run short, but I *didn't* experience that in all of that period. Now I haven't floated in more than two weeks, and I *do* experience it. Also, my stamina and endurance are *much* better, and my ease in running is much greater after floating. I don't experience any lactic acid buildup and cramping for a week or two after a float, so the effect of floating could not only be a reduction of lactic acid, but a speeding up of the clearing of lactic acid from the body."

Gmelch also noted that floating had helped him come back from injuries faster. He had frequently had problems with shin splints from his running, but he said, "I did notice that it healed quicker from being in the tank. It was quite impressive."

Float Like a Butterfly, Sting Like a Bee

Because they need to get the most out of themselves, and place such a high value on performing at the peak of their powers, athletes (along with performing artists) are constantly alert for ways of improving and maintaining their skills and tools, i.e., their bodies. Like scouts, far in advance of the rest of society, they are among the first to experiment with new approaches, trying to find practical applications for devices many non-athletes have never heard of or consider to be still in the experimental stage. But athletes usually don't care whether something is unproven or incompletely understood. Their interests are purely pragmatic: Will it work? Will it help them play better, run faster, jump higher?

Athletes were among the first to explore the practical uses of self-hypnosis, autogenic training, progressive relaxation, meditation, visualization. As for equipment, long before they were accepted as valuable by doctors, athletes were using whirlpool baths, ultrasonic treatments, biofeedback machines, orthotic devices, temporomandibular splints, and were testing, measuring, and exploring their physiological limits and potentials with sophisticated equipment such as computerized treadmills and devices to quantify strength, endurance, and speed. Since the late 1970s large numbers of professional and other top-flight athletes have begun using float tanks regularly, and the number of professional and college teams and athletes using the tanks continues to increase sharply, an indication that they are convinced the tanks work. It seems only a matter of time until tanks are as ubiquitous in training rooms, health spas, fitness centers, gyms, and athletic clubs as now are saunas, massage tables, and weight machines.

Athletes I've spoken to who have used the float tank have noticed a dramatic improvement in performance. As the brief stories above indicate, the improvement takes place on several levels, usually simultaneously, with a kind of ricochet effect, improvement on one level leading to improvement on another, and so on. Among the realms in which float tanks appear to have significant value for athletes:

≈ Increasing physical relaxation, which leads to improved performance, greater stamina, speed, strength, coordination

≈ Reduction of injuries due to overtraining or muscular tension and imbalance

≈ Alleviating the pain of injuries

≈ Enhancing the body's ability to recover from injuries and the normal stress of intensive exercise

≈ Speeding recovery from the stress of peak output (races, competition) and eliminating post-competition letdown

≈ Improved coordination and performance skills due to in-tank visualization and guided imagery rehearsal

≈ Elevating the athlete's mental state through increased confidence, concentration, calmness, and poise.

Playing Loose: Preventing Injury.   On the infinitesimal chance that someone reading this might not know a person with a sports-related injury, I should point out that such injuries are common and constitute a major segment of our national health bill. Sports-medicine specialist Dr. James Nicholas maintains records on sports injuries and has concluded that each year sports and exercise are responsible for *17 million accidents* serious enough to require a doctor's attention. "That's more casualties in one year than American troops have suffered in all our wars put together," says Nicholas.

You might assume most of these injuries are the result of naturally bruising sports like skiing or football. Jogging, for example, is a nice safe non-contact sport, right? Not so. Statistics show that while there is an 86 percent probability of injury from one season of playing football, there is an 80 percent probability of injury for a regular jogger or runner over the period of a year. Dr. Mel Thrash, director of Ambulatory Services at Bellevue Hospitals professor of psychiatry at New York University, adviser to several sports-training and health-fitness centers, emphasizes that "the majority of those injuries are related to tension." Let me emphasize this: Most sports injuries are not contact injuries but are the result of inappropriate muscular tension; most of these injuries could have been prevented by relaxation.

The best defense against injury, then, is looseness. Most athletes start their workouts with either a series of stretching movements or a gentle jog. But the preliminary loosening thus acquired is only relative. Runners, for example, can stretch for half an hour and still have tightness in the hamstrings, calves, and lower back.

There is abundant evidence, however, that the float tank causes a major and across-the-board reduction of muscular tension. Scientists at the Chicago Medical School and University of Health Sciences, Lawrence University, the Medical College of Ohio, and elsewhere have tested muscular tension on volunteer subjects by hooking them up to EMG (electromyograph) machines, and *in every case* have found dramatic decreases in muscular tension after as little as thirty-five minutes in the tank. Significantly, they found that this reduction in tension persisted for days and even weeks. We can only speculate on the effect this could have in reducing sports-related injuries of all kinds, but surely it would be a major one. Says sports-medicine authority Thrash: "An experience in the tank helps people learn to be in tune with their own bodies. *Clearly* the tank is helpful, not just in reducing tension but in giving athletes control over their autonomic nervous system. If we could train all of our athletes in this kind of tension reduction and autonomic nervous system control, I think we would eliminate a lot of these tension-related injuries and emergency room visits."

An Ounce of Prevention, a Stitch in Time ... It's interesting that Herbie, the marathon runner, claims the tank helped him avoid injuries by making him aware of points of stress or imbalance *before* they became actual injuries. "While I was floating," he says, "there might be a feeling of heat or tightness in the back of my leg, and I'd know my hamstring was getting ready to act up again, so I'd be extra careful, keep it extra loose." This predictive/preventive effect has been noted by many floaters, and most floater-athletes I've spoken with spend a part of each float session simply paying attention to their bodies, examining any painful spots, becoming aware of tensions, rigidity, misalignments of joints, points of weakness or imbalance, and trying to counteract the stress by various techniques.

Visualization. One effective method of self-maintenance is to visualize a vibrant healing energy flowing into your body. As the glowing stream courses through your body, become aware of any place where the energy seems to focus. As you find rigidities or knots of tension, concentrate all the healing energy on that spot, bathing and saturating the area with dazzling white light, visualizing the spot as becoming deeply relaxed. Envision the energy streaming through you like a river, dissolving and washing away all tensions, and see the powerful white light filling every cell of your body with health, strength, resilience, vitality, power.

Suggestion.   Such visualizations become more effective when combined with simple affirmative suggestions, such as "I feel the energy flowing through me like a surging river, filling every cell." While the imagery has a strong influence over your visual brain, it is helpful to engage the verbal areas of the brain as well. Floating significantly enhances suggestibility, so that positive statements are accepted by the mind *as if* they were actually true.

In self-maintenance and injury-prevention, the special value of floating derives in part from the enormous increase in physical sensitivity, awareness, and internal focusing made possible by the reduced-stimulus environment of the tank. The reduction in gravity increases kinesthetic awareness, as Moshe Feldenkrais's discussion of the Weber-Fechner Law (in Chapter 4) explains. "The curare effect" was demonstrated in biofeedback experiments which showed that rats totally immobilized with curare learned control of autonomic functions far better than did those to whom the drug had not been administered. Lee DiCara pointed out that the curare effect works because the drug "helps to eliminate variability in the stimulus and to shift the animal's attention from distracting skeletal activity to the relevant visceral activity. It may be possible to facilitate visceral learning in humans by training people ... to breathe regularly, to relax, and to concentrate in an attempt to mimic the conditions produced by curarization."[60]

Floating Away from Post-Game Letdown and Fatigue

With the recent mass popularity of running, millions are now discovering what athletes have long known: that after the exhilaration of competition comes the fatigue, pain, and depression of post-game letdown. This syndrome can range from a few aches and pains and a case of the blahs on the day after, to days of fatigue and depression so severe that the athlete finds it nearly impossible to get out of bed.

Some of this sense of letdown is psychological. The track meet or game you've built up to for weeks is now over; the object of all your work and mental preparation has come and gone. Now you must point toward some other contest in the future and go through the whole training process once again. There is evidence that one or more sessions in a float tank can eliminate such minor depressions completely, in part due to the release in your body of the pleasure-creating neurochemical narcotics, and the reduction of depression-linked chemicals.

But much post-game letdown is physiological. You have pushed your body to its limits or beyond; you have stressed your entire body, depleted your supply of glycogen, filled your muscles with lactic acid. You are used up, bruised, exhausted. Your body has to carry away all the lactic acid, the waste material that has built up in your system, and all the other biochemicals associated with stress; it has to build up your weakened immune system; it has to build up the muscles and other tissues that have been damaged or broken down in the heat of competition. Depending on what sort of condition you're in, and how strenuous your game was, this process will take anywhere from a few hours to several days. And while it's going on, you will not feel at your best.

Until recently there was really no way to accelerate the process. Then athletes began using the float tank and discovered that it was nothing short of miraculous when it came to post-game recovery. Dr. Mel Thrash emphasizes that floating can "speed up the recovery process enormously. What normally takes a great long period of time—days, usually, for recovery from a marathon—the tank compresses that into a number of hours. You're giving your muscles *total rest*; they're not having to do anything. Then there are the biochemical changes: All those biogenic amines that rev you up are apparently being decreased in an accelerated manner by the tank, so you're speeding up your recovery from prolonged and vigorous effort. Floating offers a *wonderful* opportunity for the body to heal itself."

Much post-game pain and stress is in one way or another related to gravity: gravity pulling the weight of the body downward onto sprains, strains, stressed joints, and bruised muscles; gravity restricting the circulation of the body's healing fluid systems, the blood and lymph; gravity's constant pull causing our already exhausted muscles to work to keep us upright. By relieving most of the stresses of gravity, even for short periods, floating takes the weight off the strained bones, joints, and muscles, and increases the efficiency of the blood and lymph circulating through the body, carrying away waste and toxins and bringing healing materials to damaged cells.

There is a wealth of evidence that floating results not only in an increase in the secretion of healing, pain-relieving biochemicals, but also in a *decrease* of biochemicals associated with stress (and post-game letdown). Studies by Fine and Turner, of the Medical College of Ohio, have shown that a single session in the float tank results in dramatic reductions in such stress chemicals as ACTH, adrenaline, noradrenaline, and cortisol. By decreasing the levels of these chemicals in the bloodstream, floating is directly counteracting the fight-or-flight reaction and speeding recovery from stressful activity of all sorts.

Getting the Bear off Your Back. Similarly, it has long been known that one of the most immediate results of strenuous physical exercise is a rapid buildup in the body of lactic acid, a toxic by-product of glucose metabolism in *anaerobic* activity (i.e., muscular activity of such intensity that the muscles' energy requirements can't be satisfied by the body's aerobic or oxygen-efficient system). Lactic acid begins to accumulate in the muscles within a minute of peak or anaerobic effort, causing great pain, fatigue, and an almost paralyzing tightness and/or muscle cramping known by runners as The Bear, as in: "I was fifty yards from the tape when The Bear jumped on my back."

When lactic acid hangs around in your muscles after competition, the result is a general feeling of sore and aching muscles that can stay with you for hours or days. Dr. Jeffrey Gmelch, who is acquainted with lactic-acid buildup both as a neurophysiologist and a runner, explained to me that while much lactic acid is eliminated by the body within twelve hours after exercise, it can take the body as long as twenty-four to thirty-six hours to clear it totally from the system. Thus, athletes who work out every day will tend to accumulate increasingly large amounts of residual lactic acid, experienced by the body as increasing fatigue and chronic muscular tension or pain. "That's why you should have one day a week that you don't exercise," Gmelch says, "to allow that residual lactic acid to be cleared from your body." By its rapid evacuation of lactic acid, the float tank speeds the recovery process, and noticeably reduces fatigue and tension.

Recent studies also indicate that lactic acid is directly related to high levels of anxiety. In fact, studies by researchers like Donald F. Klein, director of research at the Anxiety Disorders Clinic at the New York State Psychiatric Institute at Columbia-Presbyterian Medical Center in Manhattan, show that infusions of sodium lactate are so anxiety producing that they will actually induce a panic attack in 7.5 percent of subjects with a history of such attacks.[46] Clearly, lactic-acid buildup can have a disruptive effect on the athlete's ability to think clearly, to remain cool, calm, and collected, particularly in the late stages of a game or competition when grace under pressure is so sorely needed and so hard to come by. By lowering lactic-acid levels, floating can thus have a positive effect on such qualities as nerve, leadership, strategic thinking, and mental clarity—which are not usually associated with physiology.

Recharging the Batteries. One potentially revolutionary practice I think athletes should explore is that of using frequent floats during meets that extend over long periods and require repeated effort. For example, runners, swimmers, cyclists, gymnasts, skiers, tennis players, and track-and-field athletes must compete in several events during the course of a weekend competition. Often, by the time the athlete has made it to the finals he or she is physically depleted. But a session in the tank between races, rounds, or matches can help an athlete recover by sharply and rapidly decreasing the stress-related fight-or-flight chemicals, eliminating lactic acid and other fatigue-producing toxins, and bringing the body back up to peak efficiency and strength for the next go-round. As athletes who are fresh out of the tank begin to pull down gold medals in various competitions, the advantages of floating will become clear to all. I suspect that in the next few years virtually all athletic teams will acquire their own tanks, and every field house and gymnasium will provide float tanks as standard equipment in all home and visitors' locker rooms.

Floating to Stimulate Muscle Growth

Now that the old myth that weight lifting makes you muscle-bound has been laid to rest, almost all serious athletes take hard and regular sessions on Universal or Nautilus machines or with free weights. The way weight training (and in fact all high-intensity training) works is by placing demands on the body that the body cannot immediately meet. When a muscle is worked close to its limit, the body rushes oxygen and a flood of other nutrients to the muscle tissue, and carries away the waste materials. Thus, in the period that follows high-intensity exercise, the body rebuilds the overworked muscle tissue, and in the rebuilding process the muscles become larger and stronger. However, for this rebuilding and recovery to take place, the body requires time (about forty-eight hours) and rest. If high-intensity work is undertaken again without sufficient rest, the muscle not only will not get stronger, it will deteriorate. The result of over-training is loss of muscular strength, fatigue, and sickness.

Dr. Ellington Darden, director of research for Nautilus Sports/ Medical Industries and author of numerous studies of sports physiology, stresses that "for the production of best results, exercise must *stimulate* growth and *permit* growth." The stimulation is the high-intensity training, but just as essential is a period of deep rest. "High-intensity exercise stimulates muscles to grow," according to Darden, "but the stimulated muscles actually grow when the body is resting."[55] Darden says that studies of human metabolism show that virtually *all* muscle growth and strengthening takes place during rest, within a five-to-ten-minute time period about thirty to forty hours after the stimulation occurs. The float tank, with its proven ability to enhance the body's recovery capabilities, to help speed the purging of combustion debris, to bring about total relaxation, to improve the body's circulation and the distribution of oxygen and other nutrients, can have a beneficial effect on the "permitting growth" part of the muscle-building equation, and should be a significant component of any training program that includes high-intensity exercise, whether weight training or interval training.

In the coming years, sports-medicine clinics and research labs will be determining just how much the float tank can enhance muscle growth and recovery from peak output, and exactly when the best float time is (to coincide with and enhance the body's brief growth spurt). But at this time I would suggest—and the suggestion is supported by sports physicians with whom I have discussed it—that anyone involved in a high-intensity training program would profit by alternating days of peak intensity training with days of rest, and taking an isolation tank float approximately thirty to forty hours after the high-intensity exercise. If it's not practicable to float so frequently, a float at least once a week would offer the period of deep rest and relaxation that is now seen to be essential for recovery from peak output and the stimulation of muscular growth.

Playing Fast and Loose

It's important to remember that relaxation is not just an extra: It is a major component of the actual sports process, necessary for peak performance. Bud Winter was track coach at San Jose State for more than thirty years, during which time he produced a steady stream of record-breaking athletes. Essential to his training program was his belief that "relaxation is the key to championship performance." To demonstrate this to his athletes, Winter would time them going all out in repeated sprints, then tell them to run the same distance with nine-tenths effort, keeping hands and jaw loose. The athletes would always think the second time was very slow, and would be surprised to see they'd run faster than in their all-out efforts.[100]

Winter taught his athletes to trigger the relaxation response through repetition, mantra-style, of the word *calm*. As we have seen, this relaxation response can be quickly and reliably induced by floating, which also inhibits relaxation's antagonist, the fight-or-flight response. The long-lasting relaxation response elicited by floating has a number of predictable physiological effects, among them decreases in lactic acid, blood pressure, pulse rate, and oxygen consumption. Dr. Herbert Benson has studied the effects of the relaxation response in large numbers of people and ascertained that through its use, oxygen consumption can be cut by over 16 percent in just a few minutes, while even after five hours of solid sleep, oxygen consumption is reduced by only 8 percent.[21] In sports, particularly those events in which the athlete's efficient use of oxygen is crucial, the increased supply of available oxygen that results from the relaxation-induced decrease in its consumption can lead to a kind of bonus second wind—astonishing increases in stamina, strength, speed, and energy.

Tank Training Techniques

Ideomotor Signals. One technique athletes will find useful is increasing body awareness through ideomotor response, a technique described on pages 135 and 142-143. It can be used to dig up information about yourself of which you are not consciously aware—for example, whether you are overtraining, or how much and what type of training is advisable. A runner might ask whether he or she should increase daily mileage, pace, or both, and by how much, and could receive specific answers from the subconscious mind, which is incredibly sensitive to the state of every cell, organ, tissue, and system in the body.

Tapes. Another effective way to use the tank for athletic training is to play prerecorded tape cassettes over an underwater speaker system when the floater is deeply relaxed. In addition to heightening suggestibility, floating causes the brain to shift into a theta state at the same time that the activity of the right hemisphere is stepped up, and thus allows the floater to acquire information at an enormously increased rate. All the uses of in-tank tapes explored thus far by tank researchers—to improve healing, learning, strength, confidence, and so on—are clearly applicable to athletic training.

In-Tank Video. In order to take advantage of a floater's enhanced receptivity to messages, increased visual sensitivity, and ability to learn at an accelerated rate, in combination with the power of visualization, many involved in sports training are now actively exploring the use of specially installed video screens in float tanks. While the athlete floats in a state of deep relaxation, the only image in the otherwise totally black tank is whatever is displayed on the video monitor—perhaps a new football play or films of an opponent on the field, or a montage of extraordinary plays and players in action. Many have noted the benefits of watching top athletes perform—like those tennis duffers who relax with a six-pack while they watch, say, the Wimbledon finals on TV, and then go out and play far better than usual, having soaked up skillful play through observation of masters at work. But while this "osmosis effect" works well with no conscious effort, amid the distractions of a desultory Sunday at home, it is far more effective when the viewer is soaking up the TV image in a state of deep relaxation, with total concentration and absolutely no distracting external stimuli.

One team that plans to use such training methods is the Dallas Cowboys professional football team. Bob Ward, Dallas coach in charge of conditioning, foresees a combination of image and sound, directed toward increasing both learning and athletic skills: "You're lying back in the tank," says Ward, "and looking at the best catch you've made as a receiver, and you also have the sound of the crowd to reinforce that, to make you want to do it again.... I can imagine putting together a file on running backs, the best running backs that have ever played in the NFL, and just have a guy sit back in a tank and see how a guy moves." Ward is aware that such enhanced learning works best when the player is deeply relaxed, and speculates on the future: "The ultimate would be—this is down the road—when you have electrodes on; and when you're on the proper wavelength level, the thing turns on, and when you're not, it doesn't." In fact, such equipment is now in clinical use by such biofeedback researchers as Thomas Budzynski, and could be modified for in-tank use.

At least one organization, SyberVision, is exploring many ways of improving physical performance through visual stimulation. The videotapes of repeated perfect golf or tennis swings, seen from different angles, appear to imprint the image directly into the deeper levels of the brain which control muscular coordination, in a process called muscle-memory programming. One of the creators of SyberVision, Steve DeVore, has claimed that one hour of training using the company's visual system—which does not include the use of float tanks—can have the effect of more than ten hours of training on the practice field. Many researchers believe that the combination of audio-visual techniques such as SyberVision with the dramatically enhanced learning capabilities made possible by the deep relaxation and sensory restriction of the float tank should result in previously unimagined levels of achievement. The example of place-kicker Rafael Septien is compelling.

Bob Goodman, designer and manufacturer of the Ova Tank, states flatly that the effect of this combination will revolutionize sports: "The float tank is a Nautilus machine of the mind. With the addition of a video screen, the possibilities are mind-boggling. All that's lacking now is the software."

TWENTY

FLOATING
AND THE INNER GAME

Since childhood, Donna Lucco of Houston, Texas, has been a competitive athlete: AAU swimming, high school, college, and AAU track, cycling, the marathon. Following a victory in the Galveston Marathon in 1980, she set her sights on the Boston Marathon. "I trained real real hard for Boston," she says, "but I did pretty poorly. And then after that I lost interest for a while. I was kind of burned out."

Donna turned to non-athletic pursuits, earning two B.S. degrees from the University of Houston (in anthropology and psychology), and working as a counselor at a psychiatric hospital. Then she decided to try floating, emerged from her first float "feeling fantastic," and was soon floating two or three times a week. "When I really noticed the difference is on Mondays," she says. "I work all night Sunday night, so on Mondays when I would float in the morning I'd be more capable of running in the afternoon. I'd come right from work and float for two hours instead of going to bed, and I wasn't tired."

Floating renewed Donna's athletic ambitions. In the summer of 1982 she made a coast-to-coast bicycle trip, averaging about eighty miles a day. Back in Houston, she continued floating, cycling, swimming, and running, and set her sights on a new goal—the Olympic trials in May 1984.

As she stepped up the intensity of her training, she found the tank indispensable for overcoming fatigue and avoiding injury. But the tank's greatest value for Donna, she says, has been its effects in her mind: "The tank is the perfect tool for programming and goal setting, just changing your attitudes about yourself, replacing negative thoughts with positive messages." Aware that floating enormously increases suggestibility, Donna "reprograms" herself with tapes of positive messages and guided visualizations, played to her while she floats.

A recent Harris poll shows that more than 90 million Americans—59 percent of all adults—participate regularly in some physical activity, compared with only 24 percent of the population just twenty years ago. There is a parallel rise in public interest in ways of using the mind to improve on the quality of exercise. Once you begin to take physical exercise seriously there's no way you can avoid the realization that athletics is not purely a matter of muscle, with victory to the physically gifted. It is intricately linked to mental states, including such variables as psychological barriers, mind-set, confidence, will, desire, belief, concentration, coolness, and self-image.

All 90 million of today's sometime athletes have had at least some experience with this aspect of athletics, which—with the great popularity of Timothy Gallwey's *The Inner Book of Tennis* and subsequent similar books on skiing, golf, soccer, running, and more—has come to be known as "the inner game." Those who have not experimented with the inner game themselves have certainly seen it in action, as professional baseball, basketball, and football teams and various Olympic teams hire psychologists to instruct the players in hypnosis, visualization, or meditation techniques.

It may have been noticed that when the longtime also-ran Philadelphia Eagles acquired a floatation tank in 1980, the team went on to win the NFC championship, and when they went to the Super Bowl game (their first), they took a floatation tank with them to New Orleans. The Philadelphia Phillies baseball team noticed the tank in the Eagles' training room; many of its players began floating and the Phillies went on to win their first World Series for decades.

Another team equipped with a tank is the Dallas Cowboys, and star defensive back Charlie Waters said of his use of the tank in 1981: "The young players sometimes resist these techniques, but when they see those Super Bowl rings, they change their minds. In pro football, you have to make the assumption that everybody is in great shape, everybody is fast, everybody is strong. Then the difference becomes: Who can think on his feet." And it is in the mental part of the game, according to Waters, that the tank has a telling effect.

Researchers have known for years of the enormous influence of mental events over the workings of the body. Physiologist Edmund Jacobson's experiments with visualization of physical activity and corresponding muscular contractions were conducted more than fifty years ago. Later researchers became interested in just how this connection between mental image and physical response could be put to practical use, as in the now-classic experiment with the basketball-shooting school boys. (See pages 103 and 105.) One study of dart throwing matched two groups on the basis of vividness of imagery and their initial scores—that is, they were evenly matched at the beginning. One group was told to visualize themselves throwing nothing but bull's eyes. The other group imagined themselves throwing at the center but missing. The positive group improved scores by 28 percent, while the scores of the others actually *deteriorated* by 3 percent.

Could it be, researchers wondered, that such tests were showing the results only of increased or decreased confidence"? By seeing themselves as successful and accurate dart-throwers, did the subjects gain confidence in their own abilities? A test was devised in which members of one group simply imagined their darts hitting the bull's-eye, and members of the other group visualized themselves with all their senses, feeling themselves inside their imagined bodies. While both groups visualized success and should have had the same amount of increase in confidence, tests revealed that although the group that only *visualized* success had a very slight improvement, the group that visualized *and mentally experienced* the entire physical process improved dramatically. The conclusion had to be that somehow the process of vivid visualization actually improved physical coordination and performance.

Evidence of mental image's direct-programming capability began to pour in as more and more athletes learned to apply the lessons of these experiments to their own sports. Golf has always been an intensely mental sport, but Jack Nicklaus revealed the importance of visualization in his book *Golf My Way:* "I never hit a shot, even in practice, without having a very sharp, in-focus picture of it in my head. It's like a color movie. First I 'see' the ball where I want it to finish, nice and white and sitting up high on the bright green grass. Then the scene quickly changes and I 'see' the ball going there: its path, trajectory, and shape, even its behavior on landing. Then there's a sort of fade-out, and the next scene shows me making the kind of swing that will turn the previous images into reality.[172]

Richard Suinn, head of the psychology department at the University of Colorado, has done extensive work with mental imagery. Over a decade ago he attempted a controlled experiment with the University of Colorado ski team: One half of the team went into a state of relaxation, and used mental imagery, visualizing themselves skiing over the run yard by yard, taking each turn. If they made an error they were instructed to go back and correct it mentally. The other group practiced as they normally would, without visualization. But Suinn didn't get a chance to complete the experiment; since the performance of the visualization group was so far superior to the other group, the coach selected only visualizers to ski in competition, so no comparison with the control group was possible. The team went on to enormous success. Says Suinn: "What visualization does is program the muscles. Every time you do it, you're setting up a kind of computer program. When you get to the competition, all you have to do is press the start button and your body takes over—you're along for the ride." [241] Using this "visuomotor behavior rehearsal" technique (VMBR), Suinn subsequently trained several successful Winter Olympic teams.

Clearly, visualization can improve performance dramatically. But what's particularly interesting and apposite is that in all cases where athletes have used visualization techniques, or psychologists and coaches have instructed athletes in such techniques, they have emphasized the importance of *controlling* the desired athletic performance so that it is experienced as fully as possible: by visual, auditory, tactile, and olfactory imagery, by the emotional brain and the muscles and nerves.

George Leonard, author of *The Ultimate Athlete* and himself a student of aikido, writes of visualization: "It's not simply a question of 'giving it the old college try.' 'Trying' in the ordinary sense can even be detrimental. The practice, rather, entails creating a sense of the event that is vivid and fully realized, an occasion in itself.... Whatever visual or feeling language we use, the key lies in making the occasion as real and present in the realm of intentionality and structure as in the realm of energy, matter, space, and time." [136]

Herbie the marathoner understood this instinctively as he floated in the tank, watching himself cross the finish line in Central Park, hearing the crowd, feeling the nippy breeze, smelling the hot dogs—convincing himself the scene was real. And as the test of the two groups of dart throwers indicates, the difference between simply visualizing success and intensely experiencing the entire scene and process can be the difference between defeat and victory.

However, as Suinn and other experts stress, while control and richness of mental imagery is the goal, the true key to effective imagery is deep relaxation. Suinn's visuo-motor behavior rehearsal, he points out, "can be divided simply into relaxation ... and the use of imagery for strengthening psychological or motor skills." However, Suinn has found that it is often more difficult, and takes more time, to teach the athlete to relax systematically, so that the imagery will be effective, than it does to teach the rest of the technique. The problem is that athletes, like everyone else, have little experience of true deep relaxation.

Mental imagery experts have found a direct relationship between relaxation and imagery: The more deeply relaxed one becomes, the clearer, more controllable, and more frequent is one's mental imagery. And as the hard evidence cited in Chapter 12 attests, the float tank sharply increases the production, intensity, clarity, and controllability of mental imagery. Also, floating promotes the generation of large amounts of slow theta waves, which are directly linked with the production of mental images of uncanny power and reality.

Visualization Techniques

Each athlete will want to begin by picturing in the mind's eye the skills called for in competition or training, or the specific skills most in need of improvement. Often, appropriate mental images will naturally suggest themselves—perhaps an image of a swift and graceful gazelle, of winged sandals, fists of lead, or muscles like massive ropes. Each athlete must discover for himself what imagery works best: fantasy and exaggeration for some, romantic *Chariots of Fire* slow-motion for others, gritty grunting *cinema verité* realism for others. Brief descriptions follow of several visualization techniques that athletes have found particularly useful in the float tank. Try the ones that interest you, discover which work best, and be willing to change or improvise whenever you feel the impulse. Mental images can be made even more effective by combining them with repeated positive suggestions, such as: "I am running easily, effortlessly, powerfully" or "I am always able to see the ball clearly" or "Each time I come to bat I am calm, confident, relaxed, and centered."

The Mind Movie. Since you're the director of your own internal picture show, make full use of all the potentials of film making: Take the picture from many angles; zoom in and out on the ball, the goal, your feet; in moments of particular intensity or effort go into slow motion; reward great efforts with an instant replay; if you happen to make an error, go back and erase it, run through the scene again, and do it right. Give yourself motivation: Station your true love at the finish line to embrace you; read your name in the headlines of the sports pages; visualize opening a record book and seeing that the holder of the world's record is you; watch yourself deliver a victory speech over nationwide TV as Howard Cosell makes circumlocutory inquiries about your feelings.

Role Swapping. It's helpful to free yourself now and then from habitual ways by assuming a completely different style of play. Dogged defensive players should visualize themselves as offensive hotshots; laidback players can see themselves as superaggressive. This doesn't mean that you will adopt the new style in actual competition. You are just allowing yourself to experience in your mind what it is like to play in other styles.

Mental Workout.   If you are floating before a workout, visualize yourself going through each step of the training: See yourself lifting each weight, strongly, flawlessly; see yourself doing your circuit training with extraordinary speed and endurance; see yourself working up to and beyond your normal capacity, without fatigue. This can have remarkable effects. I've been told by weightlifters that since there's no necessity of waiting or resting between sets, they can run through an entire hour's workout in a few minutes of visualizing, and that the muscle-building effect of the visualized workout seems to be just as strong as the actual workout. Since tests show that imagined actions result in genuine muscular contractions, this is quite credible, and research by sports physiologists suggests that visualized workouts can in fact increase strength.

Grace Under Pressure

All right (I hear someone say), I'm sure the tank must be a wonderful place for someone who needs to relax, but I can't afford to get too relaxed. I've got to get psyched up so I can eat my opponents alive! I've got to have that old adrenaline surging through me! I need my killer instinct!

This idea of working yourself up into a frenzy, the better to unleash your aggressive and competitive energies and mobilize all your physical powers, has a long history. The problem is it doesn't work. A flood of recent studies shows there are clear physiological reasons why athletic frenzy is counterproductive. What's entailed in getting psyched is triggering the fight-or-flight reaction, an evolutionary strategy devised by the body to mobilize us instantly in the face of a threat to our security. With the release of certain hormones, we make available extraordinary strength: very good for lifting a truck off a trapped body, tearing out someone's liver, or running like hell in mindless terror, but not so hot for the kind of clearheaded strategy, pinpoint accuracy, total concentration, and perfectly coordinated finesse required in most sports.

The fight-or-flight response is not helpful in any sport in which we want a clear head and access to the peak of our powers. There is such overwhelming evidence of this that psychologists have made it a law: the Yerkes-Dodson Law, which states that a highly aroused state is good for performing very simple tasks but not more complex ones, which are accomplished better in a state of very low arousal—i.e., while calm. Easier said than done. How do we get calm, and stay calm, in a highly charged situation such as athletic competition—or performance of any sort? Or, how do we acquire what Ernest Hemingway called "grace under pressure"?

I've cited numerous studies indicating that floatation, by triggering the relaxation response, causes lower heart and pulse rate and blood pressure, decreased muscle tension, increased blood flow to hands, feet, and stomach, decreased oxygen consumption, deeper and slower respiration, increased visual acuity, decreased levels of lactic acid in the blood and muscles, increase in various perceptual-motor abilities, increased intellectual functions such as learning, recall, and problem solving, among other effects, and that these beneficial responses to floating are quite long-lasting (in some tests certain salutary effects lingered for two to three weeks). All of these effects are directly counter to the maladaptive fight-or-flight reactions.

Turner and Fine, of the Medical College of Ohio, carefully measured all these decreases in fight-or-flight or sympathetic nervous system reactions, compared them with nervous system changes in a "relaxed" control group that did not use the float tank, and concluded that floating "alters the set points in the endocrine homeostatic mechanism so that the individual experiences a lower adrenal activation rate."[252] Other tests show that while floating reduces arousal of the sympathetic-adrenal axis, or the fight-or-flight reaction, it also leads to increased visual, tactile, and auditory sensitivity, quicker reactions, and enhanced performance of both simple and complex learning tasks. Floating, then, is conducive to the calm, unshakable, steady, centered, alert, totally concentrated state of mind that characterizes top athletes working at peak efficiency.

The value of that state of mind is not limited to sports, but produces the kind of joyous, life-enhancing energy that makes it a self-validating or *autotelic* experience. It is, in fact, what we have earlier called flow, the common ingredient of all pleasurable activity, from religion to love, sports to sex, music to philosophy. Floating, it seems, is the ideal preparation and practice for all athletes, including those at play in the fields of the Lord.

Whole Brain Play

Another way of analyzing the beneficial effects of floating on athletic performance is in terms of the specialization of the brain's hemispheres. We know that when we're playing at our best, in those wonderful moments of flow, there's a wordless but perfect synchronism between body and mind. We don't have to give orders to the body; it acts perfectly, instantaneously, as in a third baseman's reflex dive for a backhanded spear of a line shot, or a flurry of volleys between two tennis players at the net, action moving too fast for the eye or the rational mind to follow.

It's apparent that the brain's left hemisphere (verbal, sequential, analytical, relatively slow, processing details) has little to do with such moments of flow, while the right hemisphere (fast, visual, spatial, holistic, synthetic) is operating freely. Athletic excellence depends so much on the nonverbal, large-scale processing of the right hemisphere that all athletes instinctively know that the intrusion of the verbal hemisphere can bring the flow experience to a dead halt. One of the oldest tricks in sports is to cause your opponent to activate the logical/verbal left brain, as when the baseball player, watching his hot-hitting opponent in batting practice, shouts, "Hey, Willie, you're hitting good! What did you do to change your stance—bend your knees more?" Willie begins to wonder what he *is* doing, the left hemisphere swings into action, and the great slump begins.

There are so many simultaneous spatial variables involved in every moment of athletic action that, if the linear, detail-oriented left hemisphere tries to interfere, it can only end up disrupting our play. And in the liberation of the right hemisphere, the float tank can be a valuable tool for athletes. As we have seen in earlier chapters, there is extensive evidence that floatation causes the dominant verbal left hemisphere to let go its usual tight hand on the controls, allowing the often neglected or undeveloped right hemisphere to come into play. Or, as Budzynski puts it: "The right brain comes out in that float tank and says 'Whoopee'."[38]

This effect, lasting as it does for many hours or days after a float, can be maintained and carried by the athlete into the arena.

The point, of course, is not to eliminate the left brain. Logical and verbal intelligence are essential to clear thinking, to effective strategy. The third baseman would not have been in position to make his reflex diving stab if he hadn't used his logical brain to consider the game situation, the batter's ability to pull the ball, and so on. Our need is not to replace left-brain dominance with right-brain dominance, but to wrest *total* control from the left brain, to keep the left brain from trying to usurp the right brain's role, to establish a cooperation and open communication between the two, so that each hemisphere is allowed to serve its proper function. And this is exactly what the float tank does: Studies of brain waves indicate that floating has the effect of bringing the electrical rhythms of both hemispheres into a state of balance and "hypersynchrony."

Crocodile Sports and Horseplay

While the visual-spatial, large-scale, rapid processing abilities of the right hemisphere are essential to all athletic activity, the true source of athletic activity and ability lies in those deeper parts of the brain that evolved earlier— the paleomammalian or "horse brain," and the "reptile brain." These ancient parts of the brain control almost all our automatic and unconscious physical activity, have immense (though nonverbal) knowledge, handle extremely subtle mechanisms like balance, coordinate movement, and direct and focus our awareness and arousal. While the neocortex is important when we are consciously trying to learn new skills—such physical activities as riding a bike or skiing, where at first we have to *think* about what we're doing—we quickly learn to do them "without thinking," which means that the physical knowledge has been handed over to our old brain. Clearly, in most sports, where we depend on the ability to perform all sorts of complicated and difficult actions automatically, we rely on the constant and unhindered working of these deep levels of the mind (what MacLean calls the visceral mind), and when they work freely we speak of the result approvingly as body/mind unity.

These primal systems of the brain are the seat of strong and irrational drives and emotions: aggression, pleasure, ritualistic behavior, territoriality, competitiveness, social hierarchies, group or team spirit, and so on, including most of those deep impulses that are the essence of sport. Our ability and desire to play games, our enjoyment of sport, and our athletic capabilities depend on communicating effectively with these older and deeper levels of the brain.

But it is our highly developed cerebral cortex that differentiates us from the "lower" animals. Our culture emphasizes and rewards effective use of the cerebral cortex. Too often, however, the result is a devaluation or even denial of those atavistic, reptilian levels of mind. We have come up out of the muck and do not like to be reminded of it. Physically as well as mentally we suffer the curse of what MacLean calls schizophysiology: a split between the new brain, which thinks, and the older brains, which act. Even when we are trying to open ourselves to the older levels of the mind, communication is difficult, since while the neocortex tends to express itself in words, the deeper brains evolved before language and operate through primal impulses, emotions, drives, images, senses, and symbols instead of verbal concepts.

Most people who engage in sports come up against this separation, which is in effect a split between mind and body. The problem is a seeming inability or unwillingness to allow those deeper levels of the mind to operate freely. This can be seen in players who are stiff, who can "learn" a sport only by consciously and painstakingly assimilating information or lessons, who can never lose themselves totally in the game, who can never open themselves up to the full range of experience and emotion that sport can provide. Rather than trusting the body which means trusting the wordless wisdom of the deep, unconscious mind—the "cerebral" athlete tries to boss the body around:

"Keep your eye on the ball, you idiot!"

But as we saw earlier, one of the primary effects of floating is to establish an integration of the old and new layers of the brain, to improve communication between the levels, open up our consciousness to an influx of energy from the suppressed and repressed lower levels of the mind. Among the ways the float tank does this are:

≈ By increasing our sensitivity to body states, i.e., allowing the neocortex to become more aware of what the deeper levels of the brain are doing. Increased body-awareness is directly linked to increased athletic capability, and all great athletes are distinguished by extraordinary body-awareness.

≈ By increasing relaxation. (Muscular tension hinders the operation of the deep levels of the mind by making it more difficult to move the body freely.)

≈ By decreasing stress-related biochemicals in the body. (The fight-or-flight reaction places the old brain in a state of imbalance, limiting its ability to coordinate and control the body.)

≈ By making the neocortex more receptive to wordless information flowing to it from the old brain in the form of images, emotions, compulsions, and the like.

≈ By making the lower brain more receptive to directives flowing to it from the upper brain in the form of suggestions and images.

These and other indications of improved communication between the upper and lower levels of the brain have been documented by numerous scientific studies of subjects in float tanks.

Recalling Socrates' charioteering metaphor for the brain, we could say the difference between athletes with or without access to the deeper levels of mind is the difference between a chariot racer with two swift horses hitched to his vehicle and one whose horses are out to pasture somewhere: Both racers may have equal desire to win, equal skills, equally good chariots, equally powerful horses, but the one with his team in harness will win the race.

Floating on the Lifetide.   While we have been dealing here with actual levels of the physiological system known as the brain, a parallel can also be made with levels of the mind or psyche, for as we gain access through floating to the levels of the brain that are older in evolutionary terms, we also gain access to the more ancient contents and modes of consciousness, peeling away layer by layer millions of years of psychic development. Floating gives us entree to what Jung has described as the Collective Unconscious: deep "memories" which are not memories of actual events but rather the memories of our species—and more, of all the millions of years of evolution. This collective wisdom comprises that bedrock of emotions, instincts, and desires that cannot be remembered consciously, but is necessarily filtered and distorted through the mechanisms of dream, consciousness, and language and emerges transformed into certain patterns: ways in which we tend to view life, which Jung called the "archetypes." [123, 124]

Throughout the first seventy years of the century, Jung's idea of an ongoing natural process to which all living things are connected, and which consists of inherited knowledge, seemed hard for many to believe. How could memory be inherited? But with recent advancements in unraveling the mysteries of our genetic material, it is now clear that it's quite possible to inherit wisdom through the unbelievably intricate codes of the DNA molecules inside every cell. The new breakthroughs in genetics are exciting, since they offer the possibility of systematic and planned access to the contents of the collective unconscious. Biologist Lyall Watson touches on this in his treatise on the biology of the unconscious, *Lifetide:* "If Jung is right about an ongoing natural process which our personal unconscious samples four or five times each night in dreams, then there might well be other ways we can experience this flow. It may be possible for us to tap into it consciously." [257]

With this in mind, it's interesting to consider the work of Jungian psychiatrist Dr. Thaddeus Kostrubala, who noticed that strenuous exercise, extended over long periods, seemed to open people up to ordinarily unconscious or inaccessible areas of their minds. He started running and noticed that he was undergoing very rapidly the kind of changes usually associated with long periods of psychotherapy. He began conducting therapy while he and his patients were running together, and made the chastening discovery that in many cases his patients were healed more by running than by his own abilities as a psychotherapist. In his subsequent book *The Joy of Running*, Kostrubala systematized his experiences, arguing that running stimulated and revealed to the runner different layers of the psyche in a fairly consistent progression and time sequence:

≈   In the first twenty minutes the runner deals with ego concerns or self-consciousness.

≈   In the next twenty minutes or so the runner descends through the personal unconscious, resurrecting and reexamining in a new light memories and emotions from the past. With the relaxation of inhibitions, physical and mental tensions and aggression bubble to the surface, bringing with them a euphoric "runner's high."

≈   Then the runner sinks into the collective unconscious, with dreamlike archetypal images emerging spontaneously; life is often seen in mythic or symbolic terms, and perceptions are intensified.

≈   And finally (after about sixty minutes of running), the runner descends into the deepest levels of the collective unconscious, experiencing oceanic feelings, full of wordless knowledge, including behavior patterns shared with animal and pre-human ancestors.[132]

This descent-through-the-layers model of Kostrubala describes very accurately what happens in the float tank, a fact demonstrated in an intriguing experiment. Boston educator R.A. (Terry) Hunt conducted a study in which about forty volunteers floated repeatedly (for a total of nearly two hundred floats) and described their experiences immediately after each one. The descriptions were then categorized into three different "orientations":

≈   The "Physiological Orientation," in which floaters showed a concern with their bodies and physical experiences, and a "present space and time" orientation—much like the early part of the prototypical run Kostrubala describes, and much like the athlete's period of warm-up and the early parts of the game.

≈   The "Ego-Centered/Cognitive Mastery Orientation," in which floaters learned to let go and become relaxed, dealt with day-to-day events and concerns, experienced imagery and memories, had "cathartic moments" in which they released their inhibitions and poured out tensions and aggression—very much like Kostrubala's middle period of the run, the experience of the personal unconscious; and equivalent to that period in sports when the athlete is playing competently but is still uninspired, still trying to direct his play with his conscious mind. In Hunt's terms, "the *ego is attempting to master the experience in a variety of ways, each of which was chosen*"; that is, the athlete is "trying to do," to rely on discipline, effort, training.

≈   The "Transpersonal Orientation": Here, the floater has inwardly directed experiences in which, says Hunt, "there appears to be no 'I' (the *witnessing ego*) involved ... in which the *experience and the experiencer are mutually causal*: each is happening to the other ... [there is] a level of concentration that can only be described as 'doing itself.'" Hunt says common experiences are merging or communicating with some spiritual entity, or a higher level of self. This parallels that period of the run when, Kostrubala says, the runner sinks into the collective unconscious; and is the equivalent of the athlete's moments of inspired play, when he is playing "over his head," merged with the game itself, not "trying to do" but simply doing. In the float tank, as on the playing field, the person who is in this Transpersonal Orientation is deeply relaxed, even while mentally extraordinarily alert, and is both "in the present space and time" and simultaneously outside of them, or, in Hunt's words, on "the interface between the infinite and the present space and time."

Hunt concluded that floaters showed a "demonstrable trend" toward what he called the "Explorative Progression," with the subjects moving from the Physiological to the Ego-Centered/Cognitive Mastery to the Transpersonal Orientation. That is, floating does facilitate (and in many ways cause) entry to deeper (or higher) levels of the mind.[106] Other experimental studies, work by psychologists and psychiatrists who use the tank for therapy, and a wealth of anecdotal evidence as well, confirm Hunt's conclusions.

For athletes, this is important news. The tank takes us rapidly, consistently, and dependably into that mental-physical state which is most conducive to peak play, to transcending ourselves. By doing so it allows us to familiarize ourselves with the physical and mental characteristics of that state, so we can reproduce them with more skill and confidence when we are actually engaged in sport. Through use of the tank we can "practice" the experience of peak play; strengthen and develop our powers of relaxed concentration, calm alertness, and effortless doing; and increase our openness to the integrative powers of the collective unconscious. And, since physiological research shows that the effects of the tank carry over for many hours and even days, we can use the tank as a preparation for athletic play, as a sort of warm-up tool to put us into a state of mind/body unity, with increased abilities of sensory discrimination, enhanced communication between the levels of the physical brain, increased access to our own too often dormant power, strength, coordination, skill, wisdom, stamina, speed.

Whether we're dealing with the lateralization of the functions of the cerebral cortex, the evolutionary layers of the brain, or the levels of the mind, floating does—in some ways we understand and in some ways still mysterious—bring about and increase a synchronous, balanced, unified, harmonious, and potentiating relationship between all parts of the brain. Through floating we are enabled to peel away millions of years of mental and physical evolution and descend to a level of cellular awareness, the collective unconscious, the Lifetide, that sets free our most explosive, serene, and inspired athletic powers.

TWENTY-ONE

FLOATING FREE
FROM HABITS AND ADDICTIONS

Recent discoveries, especially in neurochemistry, indicate that addiction is not restricted to what are usually thought of as "addictive drugs." Addiction is simply a compulsion to continue doing some thing—whether taking a particular substance or indulging in certain behavior—combined with the occurrence of stressful withdrawal symptoms if the ingestion of the substance or the behavior pattern is suddenly ended. The addictive qualities of opiates, alcohol, and cigarettes are well known, but we now know it's just as easy to get hooked on food, work, coffee, gambling, spending, sex, chocolate, other people, religion—just about anything.

Happily, scientists have made great advances lately in identifying the mechanisms of addiction. Biochemists have found, for example, that addiction is a result of changes in the body's ability to experience pleasure, its "reward system"—changes in the number and activity of the opiate receptors of the nerve cells, and in the levels of the body's internally produced opiates, the endorphins. It is also now known that the symptoms of withdrawal are associated with sudden oversupplies of the neurochemical norepinephrine in the limbic system, and that drugs that block the action of norepinephrine alleviate the symptoms of withdrawal. Such discoveries give scientists hope that they will soon develop chemical ways of overcoming addiction.

Taking a different angle of approach, behavioral and cognitive therapists and researchers have recently developed highly effective methods of attacking addictive mental processes and behavior, and it now seems clear that all who have a serious commitment to overcoming their addiction can do so, provided they follow some of the techniques for behavioral control.

Generally the worlds of the behavioral/cognitive therapists and the neurochemists are far apart, one group trying to change the imperfect actions and ideas of imperfect people in an imperfect world, the other exploring, mapping, and "correcting" microscopic electrochemical processes in the nervous system. With two completely different world views, these groups rarely agree on much. So it's significant that both behavioral/cognitive psychologists and neuroscientists now agree that the floatation tank is a powerful tool for over-coming addictions, both by changing addictive behavior and personality characteristics, and by bringing about rapid and striking changes in human biochemistry.

Smoking Cessation.   In a series of carefully controlled studies of the effects of Restricted Environmental Stimulation Therapy (REST) in the cessation of smoking, conducted over many years, Dr. Peter Suedfeld found that the effect of sensory deprivation is powerful and unprecedented. In his first study of smoking and sensory deprivation, Suedfeld claims he had little faith that REST could actually change ingrained behavior. But when he did a three-month follow-up comparing people who had undergone sensory deprivation with those who had received similar anti-smoking treatment but *without* the isolation chamber: "Lo and behold, we found that those groups in sensory deprivation were smoking almost 40 percent less than the others. This was very encouraging and very surprising."[238]

The Maintenance Effect.   A further follow-up study two years after the treat-ment found that those who had undergone the REST were still smoking far less than those who had received the same treatment without it. This led Suedfeld to the realization that sensory deprivation has a unique "mainte-nance effect." "The problem," he told me, "is not to get people to quit smok-ing, but to get them to *stay* that way once they've done it." Suedfeld's studies, and others which have followed, show that while most forms of treatment have fairly similar success rates in the initial days after treatment—when peo-ple are still highly motivated most methods quickly lose their effectiveness. But the sensory deprivation treatment maintains its power as the months, and the years, pass. Somehow, sensory deprivation makes a long-lasting change in the mind and behavior of the subject.

In his studies, Suedfeld tried sensory deprivation both by itself and in combination with a "behavioral package," including counseling and guid-ance, and found that "the combination [of the behavioral package with the sensory deprivation] is much better than either of the others. In fact, *it's bet-ter than the effects of the other two put together!* And it's close to *double* what you tend to get with the standard kinds of clinical approaches—a wide variety of behavioral, cognitive, group therapy and so forth."

Suedfeld's technique includes the playing of taped messages about the dangers of smoking, and about the subject's ability to quit smoking while the subject is in the isolation chamber or float tank. (Suedfeld has in recent years begun working with tanks.) Interestingly, however, simple sensory deprivation environment, without any messages whatsoever, also is extremely successful in changing unwanted behavior says Suedfeld, "The real problem smokers have is not in changing their attitudes, it's in unfreezing the belief-attitude-habit structure. And as I say, REST in itself, by itself, without any messages, or anything else, unfreezes that. Then the changing comes from the person's own desire to quit. Now the messages can help that, make it easier, but it can happen without messages. We have evidence for that."

Weight Reduction. One of Suedfeld's associates at the University of British Columbia, psychologist Dr. Rod Borrie, decided to apply Suedfeld's methods to what he told me was "a problem that was even harder than smoking to solve or to deal with: getting people to lose weight." Smoking, he pointed out, is a relatively simple "all or nothing" behavior pattern, while overeating is very complex. "So I took the design from some of Peter's research," Borrie said, "putting together a bunch of messages, using sensory deprivation and so on, and the results were very good."

Very good indeed: Borrie's figures show that those subjects who underwent the sensory deprivation session and received the weight-reduction messages Borrie prepared were able to lose an average of about twelve pounds over the next six months, while those who equally determined to lose weight, but only listened to the messages, or only underwent the sensory deprivation, had lost virtually no weight after six months.

But the most striking aspect of Borrie's study is that the people who combined the sensory deprivation with messages *continued* to lose weight steadily, month after month, and were still losing after six months when the study was completed. In fact, in the last four months of the six-month study period, the sensory deprivation group lost about 3.5 pounds while the other groups *gained* some 2.2 pounds. And amazingly, this continuous and extended weight loss was the result of only one session of REST. Here again is powerful proof of the "maintenance effect."[31]

In succeeding clinical studies, Borrie modified the technique by personalizing the taped messages played to the subjects in the REST environment, and found that the results were even more impressive, with some of the subjects losing as much as sixty pounds within two months.

Alcohol Reduction. Similarly successful results have been obtained in using the tank to help heavy drinkers reduce their alcohol intake, or stop drinking altogether.

While much of this work has been done using sensory deprivation chambers, many researchers (including Suedfeld and Borrie) have now begun using the float tank instead, and early results show that the tank is as effective as the chamber. In fact, there are some indications that the tank can be an even better behavior-modification device than the chamber. Certainly it is far more practical (the chamber requires a twenty-four-hour period of isolation, the tank only one hour), more enjoyable, and more easily adaptable to clinical use, private therapy, and personal behavior-modification programs.

For example, St. Elizabeth Hospital in Appleton, Wisconsin, has for several years used a float tank as an integral part of its hospital-based stress management program. In a statistical analysis of eighty-seven outpatients gathered over a one-year period in 1981-1982, the hospital noted that those who used the tank had a 50 percent reduction in cigarette smoking and a 45 percent reduction in alcohol consumption. These statistics are striking, since the program was directed at general stress reduction and not specifically toward modifying a single behavior, such as smoking or drinking.

In 1983, having moved to New York City, Rod Borne began using the float tank to assist his patients in smoking cessation, weight reduction, and a wide range of other problems. Preliminary results show the float technique to be as successful as Borrie had hoped. The tank is more effective than the REST chamber, according to Borne, because people can use the tank as a self-assessment tool to devise their own programs: "The first time in the tank," he says, "you can even work on coming up with the solutions, what you want to say to yourself *in* the tank, which is in itself very very therapeutic." And each session that follows becomes a kind of booster session, adding power to the suggestions you have already incorporated into your life. Also, Borrie points out, for the taped messages and self-suggestions to have the desired effect—the effect that causes them still to have power after six months or even two years—deep relaxation is absolutely essential. But because so few people have ever experienced deep relaxation, or know how to go about relaxing, Borrie found that he had to devote a large part of the time allotted for taped messages during his REST sessions to lengthy suggestions aimed at inducing progressive relaxation. The float tank, on the other hand, allows the subject to go rapidly and easily to a deeply relaxed state, so the behavior modification program can have its greatest effect.

Once again, then, we come to the power of the tank to combine a truly deep level of relaxation with an increase in physical and mental sensitivity and awareness. And what's intriguing is that the long-lasting stress relief and increased awareness seem often to result in reduction in addictive behavior even in floaters who were unaware of a desire for change, or who had no immediate plans to change.

Spontaneous Change

"I've always been overweight," Alice told me, "and I've tried just about everything and have never been able to lose much weight, or if I did lose it I could never keep it off for very long. But since I began floating I have lost a lot of weight, without even trying! I feel great. I had a party last week and everyone was coming up to me and hugging me and saying, 'Alice, you look great!' and that just never happened before." Among similar stories I've heard from floaters I've interviewed:

A professional photographer had become such a heavy user of cocaine that it was affecting his work. He began floating because it "sounded like fun, a trippy thing to do. I began coming over to float after work. Slowly I realized that I was cutting down on the toot, and it dawned on me that I really didn't feel like doing it all that much. I was really feeling good. *Who needs it?* I thought. I mean, this was completely an unexpected side effect."

An alcoholic musician began floating because he heard it helped you to hear music better. The night after his first float he had a concert and discovered he didn't need his usual drinks before he went on. His hands didn't shake (which had been a problem before), he had no stage fright, and friends told him he'd never sounded better. The more he floated the less he drank, and the last time I talked with him he had stopped drinking entirely for four months.

I have heard a number of similar stories. I've spoken with operators of commercial tank centers who have witnessed the effects of floating on thousands of people and claim that this is a very common occurrence, so common that they now have almost come to expect it. This seemingly anti-addiction quality of floating reminded me of studies by Harvard researchers Herbert Benson and R.K. Wallace, who measured the effect of meditation on the intake of alcohol, cigarettes, and other drugs among 1,862 regular meditators. They found striking decreases in the use of all drugs—in fact, the meditators had virtually eliminated most drug use, even though this was not a specific goal of their meditation.[24]

An even more significant study is that of Dr. Mohammad Shafii and associates at the University of Michigan Medical Center. They chose subjects who used drugs but were *not* meditators, and divided them into two groups, one that learned meditation and one that did not, so that they could find out whether non-meditators also cut down on the use of drugs over a period of

time. The study showed dramatic decreases in alcohol, marijuana, and cigarette use among meditators, while the control group showed little or no
change.[215, 216]

Other studies have supported these findings. Scientists cite such effects
of meditation as reduction in anxiety, blood pressure, and muscular tension,
and changes in brain wave activity, as possible causes of the reduction in these
harmful habits. Since we have already seen that the effects of floating on
these functions are the same as those of meditation, though more immediate,
intense, and much longer-lasting, I think it's safe to assume that floating also
possesses the anti-addiction effect of meditation—possibly to an even greater
degree. There is much evidence that this is so. Current information suggests
that *if you float, and do so with some regularity you will to all probability find yourself
cutting down or eliminating your use of cigarettes, alcohol, and drugs, and perhaps losing weight even with no systematic effort to do so on your part.*

Once we grant that spontaneous behavior change actually does take place
in an impressive number of cases, the question becomes *How?* A few of the
answers can be singled out.

Stimulus Hunger and Hypersuggestibility.   The behavior-modification programs used by Suedfeld, Borrie, and others are based partly on the concept of
"stimulus hunger." When subjects in a sensory deprivation state are presented with a taped message of suggestions, they are highly receptive. As Borne
explained it to me: "The restricted environmental stimulation creates a need
for something to happen, a 'stimulus hunger.' Anything that does happen—
first of all, it has your complete attention. And it's valued more positively
when you hear it's the only thing happening, so even if it's something really
boring it becomes interesting. It's the big event of the day."

Increased Awareness of Internal States.   "Normally," says Peter Suedfeld,
"people pay primary attention to the environment. Both through the course
of the evolution of the species and in the life of individuals, you've got to put
major attention on monitoring external events. If you go through life concentrating on your internal events, a car's going to run you down very quickly, or a tiger's going to eat you, or whatever. So, given that attention is a limited resource, and since you can't pay attention to everything that's going on
around you and inside you, you tend to ignore the latter, because for the most
part what goes on inside you is less urgent. And what the tank does is get you
out of that, because there are no external problems to solve, no external dangers to attend to. There are also no external positive rewards to strive for...."

You know, externality isn't there. So, that information processing system is free to turn inward and start monitoring what's going on inside. And you become much more sensitive, both to psychological events and to physiological events." While many people don't pay much attention to just how smoking really makes them feel, to just how much of an effort it is to carry around twenty-five or fifty extra pounds, in the float tank, says Suedfeld, "you become much more aware of how your body feels, what your internal states are. And you're *much more motivated to do something about it!*

Increased Production of Pain-Relieving, Pleasure-Creating Chemicals. Floating apparently increases the amount of endorphins in the body. This is important because there is now evidence that, in the words of Dr. William Regelson of the Medical College of Virginia: "It is very likely ... that all activities vital to survival—from sex to physical exercise—are physiologically addictive." Not just drugs, not just cigarettes or alcohol or other substances ordinarily thought to be addictive, but *all basic human drives* can be addictive.

Neuroscientist Candace Pert has pointed out:

> If you were designing a robot vehicle to walk into the future and survive, as God was when He was designing human beings, you'd wire it up so that behavior that would ensure the survival of that species—like sex or eating—would be naturally reinforcing. Behavior is modifiable, and it is controlled by the anticipation of pain or pleasure, punishment or reward. And the anticipation of pain or pleasure has to be coded in the brain. ... Emotions have biochemical correlates. ... Larry Stein, at the University of California at Irvine, has suggested that the natural opiates are the brain's own internal reward system. It seems that when humans engage in various activities, neurojuices associated either with pleasure or with pain are released.[102]

To make sure we eat, for example, our bodies reward us by releasing pleasure drugs when we eat.

A quicker way to get pleasure is to ingest some substance, such as an external opiate that fits into the opiate receptors, or a substance like alcohol, which works by causing the brain to pour out large quantities of its supply of endorphins, *or to engage in some behavior that we know by experience will cause the brain to release endorphins.*

All people have certain behavior patterns they know will bring them pleasure—that is, release endorphins—when they are hurt or depressed or in need of a quick fix of pleasure. Many like to go shopping. Go buy a hat. Physical exercise is great—get that runner's high. Clean the house. Eat chocolate. See a movie. Make love. And so on.

Since we don't indulge in them all the time, but use them only to release endorphins when we need them, most of these behaviors are fairly harmless. Some of them are even beneficial. However, there's evidence that if we overindulge in certain pleasurable activities, we can throw our pleasure/reward system out of balance. Opiate drugs do this by so flooding our opiate receptors that they shrink and diminish in number. For example, it's been discovered that the opiate methadone reduces the body's supply of endorphins so much that endorphin levels remain depressed *for six to twelve months* after methadone has been stopped. What this means is that when the external, artificial source of pleasure is removed, our own natural ability to create pleasure has withered away. We have no pleasure and no capacity to experience pleasure, and this is a very great pain that is known as withdrawal.

Habitual overeaters have no real need to eat so much. However, every few hours the pleasure chemicals in their body become depleted and they experience withdrawal symptoms. Every twenty minutes or so smokers reach for their pockets to pull out a cigarette. If they can't have a smoke they begin to get jittery, agitated, and feel the onset of withdrawal symptoms. This same pleasure-chemical release pattern holds true for all habitual/addictive behaviors, from the need to gamble to an inability to stop working.

One way to end habitual or addictive behavior patterns is to find an alternative way of stimulating pleasure. This is roughly what smokers do who take up chewing gum, or junkies who kick heroin only to turn to wine. The problem is that often the alternative routes to pleasure are almost as harmful as the addictions, not very reliable, and usually not as satisfying.

One answer could be the float tank. By providing a reliable means of activating our pleasure pathways, floating is useful in a number of ways.

Withdrawal.   In the period immediately after quitting a habit, the tank alleviates the pains of withdrawal and enables the user to feel some pleasure. Floating also reduces the level of such anxiety-related biochemicals as norepinephrine, which are released in great quantities during withdrawal. David Tenerowicz, who runs tank centers in Princeton, New Jersey, and Philadelphia, is one of a number of commercial float tank operators who have told me that many alcoholics and drug addicts use a float in the tank to relieve the anxiety and tremors of withdrawal. Tod Frueh of Tranquility Tanks in New York says that many who use cocaine have found that a float is

a good way to come down from the cocaine high: A session in the tank alleviates some of the depression and anxiety usually associated with "crashing" or
cutting off consumption of the drug after a period of use.

Post-Withdrawal.   One reason addicts find it so hard to keep from returning
to their habit even after they've kicked the physiological effects is that in the
ensuing weeks they find their lives lacking in pleasure. Much of this, we know
now, is due to their diminished ability to secrete endorphins. Nothing is fun,
because they have no ability to experience fun. By increasing endorphins,
floating enables them to experience pleasure—often for the first time in years.
Speaking of his many regulars who are former drug addicts or alcoholics,
David Tenerowicz says, "They tell me that floating lets them feel good. It
puts pleasure back in their lives, during the days and weeks after they float.
In fact, some of them felt so good they wondered at first if they could become
addicted to floating."

Assured Alternate Pleasure.   Even long after we have quit an addictive behavior pattern, there are circumstances that will cause us to want to return to the
addiction: stress, anxiety, depression, a certain individual, whatever. Usually
we can feel the pressure building, which gives us an opportunity to take pre-
ventive measures. The float tank provides an ideal escape, a pressure valve.
When we know we want to return to our addictive behavior, we can simply
take a float, stimulate our pleasure pathways, and avert the return to the
habit.

Anxiety Reduction.   Anxiety plays an important role in the formation, triggering, or continuation of addictive or habitual behavior. Floating has been
found to decrease anxiety sharply, by reducing the level of anxiety-related
chemicals in the blood, lessening muscular tension, and increasing feelings of
wholeness, confidence, competence, and security. By alleviating anxiety,
floating directly reduces the need to resort to the harmful anxiety-reduction
behaviors of smoking, drinking, eating, and so on.

Cleansing the Doors of Perception.   A vacation from normal consciousness
while in the tank enables us to return and find that, behold, everything
looks better! Like drugs, and like other meditative/concentrative techniques, floating shuts down our awareness of external stimuli, so that when
we experience them again we see them as if we've awakened from the deep
sleep of ordinary life—we have become "deautomatized." Since we can do

this safely and reliably in the tank, there is little reason to rely on more dangerous and harmful consciousness-altering techniques.

All these factors combine to help bring about spontaneous changes in habitual or addictive behavior. And they can be used by floaters consciously and systematically to change unwanted behavior patterns permanently.

TWENTY-TWO

FLOATING
FOR WEIGHT LOSS

This chapter details specific ways of using the float tank to help lose unwanted pounds. However, since all types of habitual or addictive behavior operate by similar neurochemical and behavioral mechanisms, the techniques discussed here for losing weight are applicable to all other self-destructive or harmful behavior patterns.

The Exploratory Float
The first step toward changing behavior is simply to go for a float. No matter what else happens, the float will deeply relax you. Relaxation is in itself beneficial, working to reestablish psychological balance and physiological homeostasis, with optimal levels of hormones and neurotransmitters. Relaxation not only relieves the stress that causes unwanted behavior, but also increases self-awareness.

Body Awareness.   Once you have become relaxed, focus on your body, and become aware of the effect your overeating has had on it. Are you tired? Achy? Do you have sore feet? Consider how carrying around extra pounds uses energy, puts stress on every part of your body. The more intense your physical awareness, the more powerful and long-lasting will be your motivation to do something about it.

Emotional Awareness.   At some point your attention will turn inward, your sharply focused awareness moving from your physical state to your mental state. How do you feel? What have you been feeling lately? How are your feelings related to your problem? Does the fact that you are overweight make you feel sad in certain situations? angry? guilty? For the time being, don't worry about changing anything, just become as intensely aware as possible of how your behavioral problem is linked to your mental state. The clearer your understanding of this link, the longer it will remain with you after you emerge from the tank, and the more likely you will be to try to correct the situation.

Dr. Rod Borrie, who uses float tanks to help his clients change behavior patterns, told me of how increased self-awareness helped one client lose weight: "He was in a very stressful period, both at work and at home, the very kinds of situations that usually triggered his eating, and yet he continued to lose weight. He came to me with some surprise and said, 'Ordinarily, I would be stuffing myself under this kind of pressure, but each time I get the urge to eat I become keenly aware of how this is related to my feelings, and I'm able to resist.'" That kind of continuing self-awareness is, in part, the key to the maintenance effect of behavioral change through floatation.

Self-Analysis.   With the understanding that you are now ready to solve your specific problem, begin to examine it, analyzing it, searching for its causes, its effects. When did you first begin to have this problem? What were the specific events in your life that contributed to it? Think of genetic factors, personal and family history, your current situation. Probably the most effective way to use the tank for self-analysis is to focus on your specific problem, then relax, let go, and allow your mind to find its own way. As you sink into the reverie of the theta state, it's as if your subconscious mind were on automatic pilot, it tosses up fragments of memory, faces, ideas, words. Only later do the pieces fall into place, and you see that the seemingly pointless childhood memory was actually a significant moment that has influenced your behavior ever since, that while you floated the wisdom of your subconscious mind was working creatively to help you confront and deal with your problem.

Discover Trigger Mechanisms.   Addictive and habitual behavior patterns are generally set off and perpetuated by certain environmental stimuli, conflicts, or life pressures. These trigger mechanisms are usually predictable and repetitive, and if we can become acutely aware of them, they can become signals that we are in danger of acting habitually or addictively, and we can then take action to resist the addiction. While floating, we can examine behavior patterns, see ourselves in action, search the past, and identify our personal triggers. Some common triggers are loneliness, boredom, depression, fear, a life crisis, failure, financial pressure, sexual dysfunction, fatigue, and exposure to others who share the addiction.

Understand Motivations and Expectations.   In their study of REST weight reduction, Borrie and Suedfeld made the interesting discovery that one of the

most significant predictors of success was motivation. "The motivational predictor," they emphasized, "was the importance of pleasing one's spouse. The
implication is that when one is trying to lose weight for the sake of someone
else, even someone very close, there is a poorer chance of succeeding.... In order
for the person to have the greatest likelihood of success in losing weight, she
must want to do it for herself." Everybody you know can tell you how important it is for you to lose weight, but unless you truly want to do it yourself, for
yourself, you will probably not be successful.

The other significant predictor of successful weight loss Borne and Suedfeld
isolated from their statistical analysis was that of expectation: "The expectation
variable that predicted weight loss was the amount of difficulty that the subject
anticipated she would have in sticking to the program.... Those who felt it
would be difficult lost more weight than those who thought it would be easier.... Losing weight is hard work and progress is often disappointing. An early
realization of these facts helps one to deal with them. On the other hand, unre-
alistic expectations of an easy or 'magical' solution lead to poor progress."[31]

Keeping these ideas in mind as you float, examine your own motives and
expectations. If you really do want to break that habit, are aware that you will
truly have to make an effort, and are willing to make the effort, then your
chances of success are very good.

Setting Goals.   Once you have begun to develop your awareness of the causes
and nature of your problem, and have determined your motivation and expectations, you can begin to make plans to do something about the problem. If
you are overweight, how much weight do you want to lose? Do you want to
become thin or simply lose ten pounds? The more specifically you can define
your goals, the more likely you are to attain them.

Making Plans.   You know now that you want to lose weight, and you have a
pretty good idea why; the next question is: How? You have already examined
your trigger mechanisms in general. Now watch how they work in specific situations: environmental (talking on the phone, watching TV, going to a party),
emotional (loneliness, anger, depression, anxiety), mental (self-defeating
thoughts, mental excuses for indulging, self-sabotaging scripts such as "I'm
just a fat person at heart"), and specific people (eating or drinking buddies,
mothers who insist you eat "one more helping"). Now that you're aware of the
specific circumstances that cause your habitual behavior, make plans to avoid
those circumstances, or mentally prepare responses so that you will be able to
deal with each situation without falling back on the habitual behavior. Make a

clear, systematic plan for your life: From the moment you get out of bed until the time you fall asleep at night, specify how much you are going to eat, when you are going to eat, when you are *not* going to eat.

This kind of self-exploration is an essential first step toward changing your behavior. However, self-analysis is a never-ending labor, and as soon as possible—perhaps even in your first float—you will want to go beyond self-exploration to self-transformation.

Changing Yourself

The process of actually changing the way you act and think is, of course, the heart of the matter. We have discussed it in earlier chapters under names like unfreezing, changing, and refreezing belief structures; deautomatization; and hypersuggestibility. As we have seen, numerous studies suggest that the float tank is the best tool yet devised for bringing about this transformation of attitude and action. The studies indicate that even people who are normally unreceptive to techniques like self-hypnosis become extremely susceptible to suggestion while in the tank. Suggestions given to someone in the deeply relaxed state of floating are accepted by the subconscious mind and retain their power for weeks, months, even years. (Studies by Suedfeld show a continuing effect more than two years after a single session of restricted environmental stimulation therapy.)

After you have reached a state of deep relaxation, offer yourself positive, forceful suggestions (see the section on suggestions in Chapter Seventeen). The form and content of these suggestions will depend on the self-exploration and self-analysis you have done earlier, and will consist of two different types: general suggestions directed at changing harmful belief and behavioral patterns, and specific suggestions directed toward putting your predetermined plan into action.

General Suggestions   Depending on what personal needs your self-analysis has revealed, you might offer yourself such suggestions as: You have great will power; you are quite capable of dealing with various emotional situations without falling back on habitual behavior patterns; you are filled with power and health; you are radiant with divine energy or the grace of God.

Specific Suggestions.   Make suggestions to yourself about specific attitudes and behaviors you want to change. You might tell yourself you will eat certain foods that are good for you; you will increase your energy expenditure by walking up and down stairs; you will limit your food intake in certain ways, such as eating in only one predetermined place, eating very slowly, not eating while watching TV; you will act to increase your awareness of the consequences of eating, perhaps by keeping a daily record of calories, weight, and so on.

Visualization.   The more clearly you can see an action or situation in your mind's eye, the more strongly it will tend to become real. As you float, and in conjunction with the suggestions, visualize yourself acting as you want to act. If you are trying to lose weight, hold an image of yourself as you would like to be: slender, with skin taut and smooth, waist narrow, glowing with vitality. Imagine yourself in situations that usually trigger your habitual behavior, and visualize yourself resisting.

Addictive activities cause us to release pleasurable neurochemicals, and one of the difficulties of quitting is that we are left with a limited ability to experience pleasure. So, in addition to visualizing moments in which you resist your habitual behavior, also visualize vivid scenes in which your habit plays no part at all—scenes of yourself living a vigorous, happy, fulfilling life without your habit. This kind of visualization seems to work in several ways: The subconscious mind tends to accept vividly imagined scenes as real, and therefore the visualized behavior can, through repetition, become grooved into your mind as powerfully as if you had actually lived it. Also, since the scene is accepted as real, if you see yourself experiencing pleasurable emotions, your brain will automatically respond by releasing neurochemicals such as endorphins, with the result that you immediately feel very good even as you are floating. These feelings will stay with you, and will help you avoid returning to your habitual behavior.

Tape Recordings   Playing tapes is even more effective than giving yourself suggestions, since while you're floating you have a tendency to become so relaxed that getting organized enough to give yourself a systematic series of suggestions seems to demand immense effort. A taped message, on the other hand, seems to come from everywhere, allowing you simply to relax, accept, contemplate the suggestions being offered, and visualize their being put into action. Suggestions seem particularly effective when combined with background music. The music should be nondisruptive, stately, harmonious, light, melodious, gentle, flowing.

After an exploratory float or two, in which you find out what behavior you want to change, and how to go about achieving that change, write out your suggestions—positive, concrete, vivid—and read them onto the tape as the music plays in the background. Or you might want to have them read by someone whose authority you respect, or whom you love. Read confidently, with feeling. Leave pauses between suggestions—this gives you time to ponder them and to visualize their results. Probably fifteen to twenty minutes of tape are sufficient.

Anyone using the float tank in a systematic program to break a habit will want to schedule floats regularly—at least once every two weeks, more frequently if possible. However, if at any point you are under particular stress, or feel that one of your trigger mechanisms has been activated, you can short-circuit the process with a float. By removing you from stress, relaxing you, giving you pleasure, and enhancing your ability to experience pleasure in everyday life, the float will remove or lessen your need to experience pleasure through your habitual harmful behavior.

TWENTY-THREE

FLOATING AWAY
FROM DEPRESSION, ANXIETY
AND FEAR

At this point it should not surprise you to discover that mental states like depression and anxiety are associated with very specific biochemical secretions, or that going into a float tank has a dramatic effect on the biochemicals associated with depression and anxiety. This makes sense, since the place where external events—such as a divorce or an airplane flight—are translated into physiological/internal events is in the visceral brain, particularly through the actions of the hypothalamus and pituitary; and it is in exactly that part of the brain that the experience and sensation of floating in an isolation tank has its most direct influence.

Depression
We have discussed at some length the stress reaction known as the fight-or-flight response. Far back in evolutionary history, animals developed the ability to deal with a threat to their security by activating the sympathetic system, thus preparing themselves to fight or to flee. The sympathetic system is activated through a rapid secretion of catecholamines (i.e., epinephrine, norepinephrine, and dopamine). However, scientists have recently come to believe that during recent evolution a new reaction has been added to the catecholamine fight-or-flight response—a "third way," which involves the release of ACTH and cortisol, and has been necessitated by the complex social environment in which higher animals must live, where neither fighting nor active flight is a practical option. This alternative to fight or flight is described by Dr. James Henry of the Department of Physiology and Biophysics, University of Southern California School of Medicine:

> In the ethological context, the ACTH-corticosterone mechanism is involved when the decision is made not to respond to challenge with fight or flight but to pursue this third alternative. In a social situation in which there is a hierarchy with a single dominant or an establishment group in control, this third option is of utmost importance. It

involves submitting to the demands of the dominant animal or to the establishment and involves inhibiting previous patterns of behavior. When there is conflict instead of aggression or flight ... the individual may gain much by submission and by experiencing depression associated with the loss of control. The depressed animal with high ACTH no longer competes but accepts the unpleasantness of frustration.[98]

Humans are clearly the supreme example of animals living in a highly evolved and complex social situation, often with both a single dominant animal (such as the boss) and an establishment group in control. Humans are also frequently unable to give in to aggression or flight, and must accept internal conflict and the unpleasantness of frustration; for example, the fight-or-flight response is of no use when the boss tells you your job is on the line. Humans may gain much by this submission, but they also experience frequent bouts of the depression, and the elevated levels of such biochemicals as ACTH and cortisol, that go along with it.

Many recent studies have shown, in Dr. Henry's words, that "helplessness is a crucial determinant of depression. Individuals who are most vulnerable to depression and who show the greatest response are those who find that their efforts to cope are consistently failing." Helplessness has been demonstrated in a number of laboratory studies to lead to a great rise in plasma cortisol. On the other hand, tests have also determined that while submission and helplessness are associated with elevated ACTH and cortisol, dominance and confidence are associated with lower baseline cortisol values.

Numerous studies have established conclusively that depression is associated with higher levels of cortisol and ACTH. There is also overwhelming evidence that humans who exhibit Type A behavior (aggressive, competitive, struggling against time) are more susceptible to depression under stress, and also reveal abnormally high levels of cortisol and ACTH. Also, as Dr. Henry points out, in a recent study by Earl Ursin of humans subjected to stressful situations: "Cortisol correlated negatively with performance and positively with fear and was related to the Freudian defense pattern. Ursin perceived a relationship between cortical hormone and specific psychopathological processes, i.e., depression and defective immune response mechanisms." [98]

These consistent linkings of depression with elevated pituitary-adrenal activity (i.e., plasma cortisol and ACTH) are striking and important. Float tank researchers John Turner and Thomas Fine have measured the effects of floating on these chemicals: Testing two groups over eight sessions, Fine and Turner found significant decreases in plasma cortisol and plasma ACTH among the floaters. "We also saw," says Turner, "that the REST group maintained this reduction in cortisol over a five-day period after the floating. That is, five days after their last float, their plasma cortisol levels were still significantly below their baseline and significantly below the control levels." Among their conclusions: Floating is "associated with specific decreases in pituitary-adrenal activity."[252]

So, completing the links: Depression is associated with helplessness and submission, and all three are linked to elevated levels of pituitary-adrenal activity. Floating causes dramatic and long-term decreases in pituitary-adrenal activity. The equation is clear: By sharply reducing the biochemicals associated with depression, floating should reduce or alleviate depression. I say "should" because no one has yet done a controlled study of the specific effect of floating on depression, but it seems apparent that at least in the types of depression linked with helplessness and elevated ACTH and cortisol, the effect of floating must be decidedly beneficial. A number of controlled studies in which subjects were evaluated as to mood and emotion demonstrated that floaters experienced a definite elevation in mood and an increased feeling of well-being. (The type of depression we are dealing with here is the common sort caused by life stresses and events. This does not include the most severe types of depression caused by genetic or other long-term biochemical imbalances. Indications are that these severe biochemical depressions are not helped by floating.)

But while there have as yet been no rigorous scientific studies of floating and depression, there is much anecdotal evidence that floating is an effective way to eliminate or alleviate depression. If depression is consistently linked with helplessness and submission, floating has been consistently linked with feelings of control, coping, and dominance. (As noted above, dominance is linked to lower levels of cortisol, and floating decreases cortisol.)

Other behavioral symptoms linked to depression include insomnia, dread, loss of appetite, loss of interest in sex, difficulty in concentrating, fatigue, suicidal thoughts, feelings of hopelessness. In my interviews with floaters, and in the experience of float center operators and medical professionals who use float tanks, the normal response to floating is the opposite of these depression symptoms: increased interest and pleasure in sex, better sleep, increased sensory enjoyment, clearer and more effective thinking, increased vigor and gusto, feelings of optimism. This evidence is compelling but not scientifically conclusive, since it does not come from controlled studies of depression sufferers. However, in studies using a sensory deprivation chamber, Canadian researchers H. Azima and F.J. Cramer placed psychiatric patients in the chamber for periods of from two to six days (the length depending on the patients' own wishes and responses) and found the symptoms of depression sufferers dramatically improved.[7] As described by Princeton psychologist Patricia Carrington: "This improvement lasted after they came out of the isolation chamber and did not disappear. These patients now showed greater motivation, more socialization with other patients, and great self-assertiveness. Some of them responded so well to sensory isolation, in fact, that they improved to the point of being discharged from the hospital. This was particularly interesting in light of the fact that some of those who could be discharged in this manner had been long-standing chronic 'incurable' hospitalized patients."[45]

Anxiety

Tight chest, sweaty palms, pounding heart, dread, feelings of loss of control or impending panic, butterflies in the stomach, irritability, restlessness, trembling hands, fear, a sense of foreboding—we have all experienced one or more of these symptoms of anxiety. In many cases anxiety is an appropriate response to a specific threat. But when it spirals out of control into panic, or is not associated with a specific cause or object and becomes a chronic "free-floating" anxiety, or is irrationally triggered by some specific object or situation and becomes a phobia, anxiety is a life-disrupting, debilitating illness. It is an illness that seems to have reached epidemic proportions in our culture.

Like depression, anxiety is an illness with specific physical and hormonal effects, including muscular tension, elevated blood pressure, heart rate, and pulse; and extremely high levels of norepinephrine, epinephrine, and cortisol. Numerous controlled studies of the physiological effects of floating have proved conclusively that it reduces muscular tension, blood pressure, heart rate, and pulse (e.g., O'Leary and Heilbronner;[176] Stanley, Francis, and Berres;[228] Belden and Jacobs[19]), and studies by Fine and Turner have shown significant decreases in the anxiety-related biochemicals. Another significant contributor to anxiety is lactic acid; laboratory and clinical tests show that an infusion (slow injection) of this chemical into the bloodstream will cause intense anxiety and panic attacks in 75 percent of those with a history of anxiety problems. Floating's ability to lower lactic acid must have powerful anxiety-relief or anxiety-prevention effects. Studies in which subjects were evaluated for anxiety (e.g., O'Leary and Heilbronner) have shown that floating decreases subjective feelings of anxiety.

Even more impressive are the figures gathered by Dr. Allen Belden and Gregg Jacobs of St. Elizabeth Hospital, Appleton, Wisconsin. The hospital has used a float tank as part of its outpatient stress management program for several years, and psychiatrist Belden says they have found that most of the patients they have treated for various complaints have been suffering from anxiety. It is, he says, the "common key," superimposed on most other problems. In a one-year statistical study, Belden and Jacobs found that the float tank was impressive in reducing anxiety: In all subjects, floating reduced intensity of anxiety by 74 percent, frequency of anxiety by 65 percent, psychophysiological symptoms of anxiety by 65 percent.[19]

Dr. Melvin Thrash, director of Ambulatory Service at New York's Bellevue Hospital, and associate professor of psychiatry at New York University/ Bellevue Medical Center, believes that perhaps the greatest value of the float tank is its anxiety-reducing effect: "The hallmark of every psychiatric disorder is anxiety ... and that's my major interest here, the person who comes in who lives every day in terror, and the terror has no specific reasons—this vague, free-floating anxiety. If I can help that person spend an hour a day away from that terror, then I've made an inroad that will enable me to help that person divorce himself from that, and in time not be crippled by this kind of anxiety."

Thrash told me that he believes the tank "absolutely" reduces anxiety, and does so in part by increasing the floater's "sense of well-being." "Most people who are psychiatrically diagnosable are people who've never felt good about themselves; and this cycle feeds on itself. And if you can interrupt that cycle just for a couple of hours with something that allows them for once to experience what it's like to feel good, then you have something to build on."

The immense importance of the tank as a natural anti-anxiety tool can be appreciated in considering the widespread use of anti-anxiety drugs in our society. Valium and other similar drugs account for a sizable number of emergency-room incidents, along with a growing problem in addiction. The reason Valium, Librium, and related drugs known generically as benzodiazepine are so effective in relieving anxiety is that the brain has certain receptor sites into which benzodiazepine fits exactly, just as heroin fits into opiate receptors. These binding sites, discovered in 1977 and quickly dubbed "Valium receptors" by neuroscientists, indicate that the body must create its own natural anti-anxiety substances (still undiscovered), just as it creates endorphins to fit into the opiate receptors. And just as opiate receptors accept external substitutes such as heroin and morphine, but at the cost of decreasing the body's own opiates and number of opiate receptors, which can lead to addiction, so scientists now have demonstrated that excessive use of external benzodiazepine causes a diminishing of the body's own ability to counteract anxiety. Thus the addictive nature of Valium—a user's natural ability to produce an anti-anxiety neurochemical (or the number of receptor sites for such a neurochemical) atrophies, and when the user stops taking the drug, he or she will experience extremely high levels of anxiety for weeks or months, until the body can restore its innate capabilities.

Also frightening is what happens to babies born to women who are taking Valium. Neuroscientist Candace Pert has pointed out: "If you give a pregnant rat one shot of Valium, for example, its babies will have half as many Valium receptors [as normal] when they grow up. This raises frightening questions about current obstetrical practices."[102] It's possible that pregnant women who take Valium are condemning their babies to a lifetime of high levels of anxiety.

Even more frightening are the studies by Dr. David Horrobin (corroborated by Dr. Rashid Karmali of New York's Sloan Kettering Cancer Center) that rats treated with small quantities of Valium (at low dosage *comparable to a human dosage of only five milligrams per day*) developed three times as many cancerous breast tumors as did rats who did not receive Valium.[254] Statistics indicate that more than two thirds of the users of Valium are women, and the incidence of breast cancer has risen sharply in recent years. While such figures are only suggestive, there can be no doubt that anti-anxiety drugs are dangerous. We live in an anxiety-producing world, and it's imperative that we find safe ways of relieving anxiety. The existence of Valium receptors in the brain indicates that we produce our own natural anti-anxiety substance. Every test used to measure the anxiety levels of subjects before and after floating has demonstrated that floating dramatically reduces anxiety. Though it has not yet been proved, it seems probable that, just as floating apparently increases the secretion of endorphins, so it increases the secretion of the still-undiscovered natural anti-anxiety substance. And it is probable that just as we can learn to pump up our endorphin levels through conscious self-regulation in the float tank, we can learn to increase our levels of natural Valium. The float tank begins to look more and more like an essential health maintenance tool.

Phobias

Fear reactions triggered by specific objects or circumstances—dogs, snakes, high places, germs—are known as phobias. Phobias can lead to anxiety or panic, or cause the sufferer to change or limit his life to avoid the phobic trigger. Anti-depressant drugs do not help phobias. Phobic reactions seem to result from conditioning (for instance, a child attacked by a large dog may develop an irrational fear of all dogs), and using various deconditioning techniques, behavior therapists have been extremely successful in helping people overcome phobias. Probably the most effective technique, known as *systematic desensitization*, involves creating a graded hierarchy of fear-producing stimuli. Someone with a fear of snakes, for example, might list ten situations, from a not very scary number ten, such as seeing a photo of a snake, through progressively scarier ones (being in the same room with a caged snake, seeing someone else in the same room hold a snake), to the most terrifying one (holding a live snake). The subject would then begin by confronting situation number ten until it no longer held any terrors, then move on to nine, and so on, becoming progressively desensitized.

This is often combined with *reciprocal inhibition*, in which the trigger situation is paired with a counteractive calming stimulus or technique, such as muscular relaxation, visualization of a peaceful scene, or deep breathing. It has been found that if anxiety-provoking stimuli are produced in the presence of deep relaxation, they seem to lose their charge. So, while moving up the hierarchy, the subject confronts each situation, and simultaneously practices the relaxation technique, until phobic reactions disappear, with the ultimate goal of confronting the most terrifying phobic situation and remaining calm.

Clearly the float tank can be an effective tool in combining these techniques for overcoming phobias. By inducing utter relaxation, it enables the floater more quickly and easily to overcome the tension and other correlates of fear; by increasing the power of visualization, it helps the floater imagine the phobic situation more clearly and realistically, and also to imagine himself or herself overcoming the phobia and acting fearlessly in that situation; by eliminating all distractions and other external stimuli, it enables the floater to focus specifically and exclusively on confronting and overcoming the phobic situation.

"What I would really like to do is work in the tanks with people who have problems with phobic responses—using systematic desensitization," says psychiatrist Thrash. Peter Suedfeld has successfully treated snake phobia in this manner using a sensory deprivation chamber, and has begun work using the float tank for desensitization therapy.

The Tank as Psychotherapeutic Tool
In his survey of the effects of sensory deprivation, "The Benefits of Boredom," Peter Suedfeld noted that "psychiatric patients tended to relate better to their psychoanalyst after" being in sensory isolation; that "other researchers have

reported improvements in various personality test responses, body image, symptomatology, reality contact, and social interaction"; and concluded that sensory isolation influences "in one way or another, processes as various as the electrical activity of the brain, biochemical secretions, galvanic skin response, basic sensory and perceptual processes, cognition, motivation, development, group interaction, the relationship between environment and personality characteristics, learning, conformity, attitude change, introspection, and creativity. This is probably as wide a range of effects as has been investigated in any substantive area by any technique known to psychologists."[234]

We have noted the persuasive evidence that float tanks can be enormously effective in alleviating depression, anxiety, and phobias. In the light of such evidence it is hard to understand why psychiatric hospitals have not yet begun to use the float tank as a form of treatment, while they continue to rely on electroconvulsive (or shock) therapy and powerful drugs which have well-known harmful side effects. There are indications, however, that this is changing. As more and more doctors, psychiatrists, psychologists, and other health professionals become aware of the beneficial effects of floating, often through their own experiences in the tank, there is increasing pressure on hospitals to accept the efficacy of floating, and several doctors have told me that they expect that float tanks will soon become common in mental health facilities.

There are already many mental health professionals in the United States and Canada who rely on the float tank as a therapeutic tool, either by integrating it directly into the therapeutic process or, like Dr. Thrash, by recommending it to patients as an adjunct to therapy. Many traditional forms of psychotherapy have long used less effective methods of sensory deprivation. In psychoanalysis, for example, the patient reclines on a couch (to facilitate relaxation), with the analyst sitting out of sight, saying little, so that the analysand can turn attention inward and allow mental contents to surface in a process of free association. The characteristics of the float experience—deep relaxation, self-exploration through mental imagery and free association, absence of anxiety, release from tension, growth in feelings of wholeness and well-being—are exactly the characteristics most conducive to advancing the therapeutic process.

People engaged in therapy will be helped by taking a float either before or after a therapy session. "Either way," says Dr. Thrash, "would have a payoff. Hopefully, in the session you are effective enough so that you stir things up, so that going into the tank afterward would allow him to sort out a lot of questions; going in before hopefully would bring up a lot from the unconscious that you could work on in the session." Thrash also points out that the relaxation brought on by the tank would help people open up, stop "blocking," and become more aware of physical tensions related to mental problems. "The thing I like about the tank," says Thrash, "is that you do it yourself."

TWENTY-FOUR

FLOATING TO
HIGH-LEVEL WELLNESS

Humans have probably always known that the mind and body are one, dual aspects of a single reality, inextricably linked and interdependent. Certainly they have known for thousands of years that the body can be changed and controlled to a large degree by the mind, and that this can be accomplished most effectively by putting the body into a state of deep relaxation and guiding or manipulating it through vivid images—for every culture has developed its own means of reaching states of deep relaxation, its own rich and colorful array of images which it has found effective in influencing and changing the body.

Shamans and witch doctors enter trances to see themselves as hawks or coyotes, conferring with the spirits of natural forces; or, representing those spirits and forces, they dance in bright, monstrous masks before a sick person. With astonishing frequency they bring about cures. Immobilized and confronted with the proper images, the body is changed. Yogis devote years to learning how to enter states of deep relaxation at will, and when in that trance they visualize energy flowing up and down the moon channel, the sun channel, flooding various centers of force known as *chakras*, which are themselves seen in images as points of certain vivid colors—and as a result their bodies change; they can slow or even stop their hearts and respiration, can cast off sickness. Myths, fantasies, religious ceremonies, dreams, visions, poems and psalms and hymns—all have served, to some degree, as ways of controlling and changing the human body, and have been more effective when the body is in a state of deep relaxation: trance, reverie, prayer, meditation.

However, with the development of the "modern mind" or Western civilization, the idea that mind and body were one and inseparable became suspect: a product of the childhood of our race, primitive, now outmoded and outgrown. After all, science *worked*, didn't it? The body is a machine, and how can something called mind affect a machine?

But in recent years, using its own scientific method, science has accumulated an overwhelming amount of evidence that the body is not a machine, that mind is something quite real and powerful, and that in some mysterious way the mind not only controls the physiological body but is in fact a part of it.

It was found that some hay-fever sufferers who looked at a picture of ragweed began to sneeze. Some patients, told that the pills or injections they were given would kill their pain, or cure them, immediately stopped hurting or recovered. Scientists called this the placebo effect, but that didn't disguise the fact that what was happening was much like a witch doctor dancing in a bright mask or administering empty potions that still cured illnesses.

Cancer patients were taught to become deeply relaxed and visualize their white blood cells eating and destroying the cancer cells, and an astonishing percentage of them recovered. Tests of men whose wives were dying of breast cancer showed a sharp decrease in white blood cell function; as they became depressed, their immune systems weakened. Hooked up to biofeedback machines, people could learn to change their heart rate, kidney function, release of hormones.

Somehow, purely mental states were changing what had been thought to be purely physical states: cancer cells, the immune system, the autonomic system. But until recently there has been no real explanation of how this was accomplished. Now, and only in the last few years, scientists have come to see that the mechanism through which feelings and emotions and thoughts could be translated into cancers and colds and heart attacks is the neuroendocrine system, via the release of hormones, neurotransmitters, and other biochemical substances. The place of transmutation, the alchemical laboratory where emotions and visions and ideas are made flesh and blood, is largely centered in the hypothalamus. Releasing chemicals that act on other glands like the pituitary, thymus, and adrenals, the hypothalamus can cause the release of catecholamines; neurotransmitters like the endorphins; chemicals that can raise or lower blood pressure, kill pain, bring euphoria or anxiety or rage, suppress or strengthen the immune response.

There is no doubt of this. What takes place in the mind is not separate from what takes place in the body. Biofeedback researcher Elmer Green has stated the relationship clearly: "Every change in the physiological state is accompanied by an appropriate change in the mental-emotional state, conscious or unconscious, and conversely, every change in the mental emotional state, conscious or unconscious, is accompanied by an appropriate change in the physiological state."[87]

This knowledge that our thoughts determine our physical condition has been one of the most exciting discoveries of our time, and has resulted among other things in an entirely new field of medical research called *psychoneuroimmunology*. And it has led to an even more exciting and truly revolutionary discovery: By controlling our thoughts, we can control our bodies and our health.[2]

Biofeedback taught us what yogis and shamans had known for centuries: Any biological function that can be monitored and fed back to us through our senses can be regulated by the individual. This led to the further discovery that electrical biofeedback equipment was not necessary; purely through intensifying our awareness, we can regulate our bodies. The technique is simple, and is based on thousands of years of empirical verification: A concentrated meditative state of deep relaxation leads to the establishment of voluntary control by allowing us to become acutely aware of internal sensations, images, and ideas.

The problem for our culture has been getting into the state of deep relaxation. Most people in our society are unwilling or unable to undergo the long training period required by most of the traditional techniques for quieting the body and intensifying awareness of internal states. This brings us to the floatation tank as a powerful tool for gaining and maintaining a high level of health.

Relaxation
Through all sorts of tests (described earlier), including EMG (which measures muscle tension), EEG, blood pressure, and measurements of certain biochemicals, scientists have determined that the float tank can bring about a state of extraordinarily deep relaxation—probably deeper than is possible by any other means yet available except for certain drugs. This state of relaxation is in itself beneficial to health, since it allows the body to maintain its internal system of checks and balances, its homeostasis. That is, the body has its own highly effective methods of maintaining itself at an optimal level of well-being, and if allowed to operate freely, it will generally do so flawlessly. But certain mental attitudes can throw this delicate mechanism out of whack. Stress causes harm by its disruption of our natural biochemistry. For example, researchers have recently discovered that, under stress, Type A personalities secrete forty times as much cortisol and three times as much adrenaline as Type B men.[103] Cortisol has been proven to suppress the immune system. Tests have shown that floating decreases cortisol. Excess adrenaline, and related biochemicals such as noradrenaline and ACTH also cause our

bodies to rev up in a fight-or-flight response, and, ultimately, to wear out. Floating, through deep relaxation, lowers the levels of these harmful chemicals.

Deep relaxation is beneficial in another way. Because of what has been called the curare effect, and as explained by the Weber-Fechner Law, floating leads to increased sensory awareness; we simply feel our bodies better, more clearly, and as a result we are able to regulate them more effectively. As John V. Basmajian's experiments showed, we have the capacity to control the firing of a single motor neuron in the body, once we are made aware of that neuron.[15]

Deep relaxation also leads to improved access to internal imagery. And awareness and control of mental imagery is the key to self-regulation.

Also, the deep relaxation of floating feels good. In part this is because of the temporary rest and release from the stresses of life. In part, there is reason to believe that floating in some way causes the body to release certain biochemicals that make us feel very good indeed—such as the endorphins and the as-yet-unidentified anti-anxiety neurochemical that fits into the "Valium receptor." Euphoria is a nice place to spend the day, but we should also remember that it is conducive to health. We know that feeling good makes us healthier; feeling whole increases our wholeness; feeling well increases our wellness.

Stressful events affect people differently. Recent tests showed that subjects who had a high level of perceived stress in response to certain life events had a greatly reduced level of immune response, only one third the level of "natural killer cell activity" of those who experienced the same life events but perceived them as less stressful. By making us feel less threatened, anxious, and stressed, floating enables us to cope with the same stressful situations that might otherwise have impaired our health.

What does this mean for us? First, the mere act of floating, in and of itself, is healthful because it is relaxing and makes us feel good. Simply by floating, even if only once every few weeks, we can strengthen our immune systems, increase our ability to withstand and respond to stress, reduce the level of harmful biochemicals in our systems, and become stronger and happier.

Second, if we are sick or have physiological problems, we can consciously use visualization and self-suggestion techniques in the tank to increase the body's healing ability. Cancer patients have cured themselves by visualizing their white blood cells as ravenous white dogs or white knights on horseback. We can use the same method for any illness or injury we wish to treat; we can visualize a broken bone healing, cut flesh knitting and becoming whole, headaches lessening and disappearing. We can do this anywhere, but the tank has been shown to be the most effective available tool for creating, manipulating, and concentrating on vivid mental imagery.

Research has also demonstrated conclusively that floating increases our suggestibility, the characteristic at the root of the placebo effect, which in a sense tricks the body into pouring out its own internal pain killers and curative powers. By changing our brain wave rhythms, by increasing access to the minor brain hemisphere, by enhancing communication between the conscious roof brain and the deeper levels of the brain, floating enables us to give ourselves verbal messages and to have those messages received, accepted, and acted upon as if they were true. All evidence now indicates that simply by floating, speaking healing and positive thoughts, and accompanying them with vivid healing imagery, we can heal ourselves.

Third, it now seems clear that we can use the tank, even if we have no injury or sickness, to pump up the body's natural immune system by visualizing our systems bathed with a flood of beneficial biochemicals, the thymus and hypothalamus and pituitary pouring out healing biochemicals, the protective white blood cells flowing through us, the subtle restorative energy streaming like a healing river of light. You may use whatever type of imagery you feel most comfortable with—one person has spoken of seeing his heart like a huge house, of walking inside it and strolling through the rooms like a carpenter, fixing it with hammer and nails and plaster. The translation from conscious impulse to body change seems to be almost immediate. In a recent study conducted at Penn State, subjects were pretested to ascertain the strength of certain measurable parts of their immune systems, and were then hypnotized. They were given the suggestion that they would visualize, and bring about an increase in the number and activity of, these parts of the immune system. In a one-hour post-hypnosis test, researchers found that the number and activity of those parts of the immune system were indeed significantly increased.[162] The implications are immense, particularly for floaters, since the tank not only makes self-hypnosis easier and stronger but also dramatically enhances suggestibility without hypnosis. What can be done with simple hypnosis can be equaled and surpassed in the tank.

A growing wealth of scientific evidence demonstrates that if we maintain our bodies at a high level of wellness, we cannot only live healthier lives but can increase our longevity. One current theory much in favor holds that aging is due to a slowly developing hormonal or neurochemical imbalance, rather than any specific alteration in a single vulnerable system: that is, aging is a slow disruption of homeostasis. There is evidence of such an "aging clock" located in the hypothalamus, with scientists detecting "significant decreases in neurotransmitter chemicals in the hypothalamus from old compared to young animals.[255] By maintaining a proper homeostatic balance of neurochemicals—which, as we have seen, is one effect of floating—it may be possible to be both healthier and longer-lived.

Neuroendocrinologist John Turner hinted at this in describing the results of tests he and Tom Fine conducted on the effects of floating on certain neurochemicals in the blood. Before the tests they took blood samples from each subject to establish what is called a baseline. They found that before the subjects had floated, there was a large variance in the levels of the various biochemicals being tested. However, as the subjects floated, and over a series of floats, this variance grew smaller and smaller. Said Turner, "Tom and I feel that this may well represent a *baseline effect* that occurs in the tank. In other words, the individual is in an environment where he's passively relaxing, his metabolic, physiological activity is coming down to a baseline, and *the individual is essentially reregulating himself at a lower level of variability.* We all know that an internal combustion engine runs much more smoothly when it's well lubricated and its tolerances are small. And if you'll allow me that analogy, I think the human body may well run much more smoothly when the variances and the tolerances are small."[252]

To continue the analogy, an engine that is well lubricated, well tuned, with small tolerances, will more efficiently, and it will last longer than an engine with loose parts and constant friction, an engine that is constantly being revved up. Like impatient drivers repeatedly gunning our engines, we flood our systems with the fight-or-flight biochemicals that keep us revved up. Floating seems to allow our bodies to regain their natural states of fine tuning—which is known as health.

How does floating affect learning ability? Texas A & M chemistry professor Dr. Thomas E. Taylor set out to answer that question in one of the most ingenious and meticulously executed studies in the history of float tank research. In the spring semester of 1982, Taylor carefully screened the EEG recordings of more than 450 volunteers to eliminate variables, and pared the group down to 40 subjects as near to identical as possible. His final group was all female (to avoid any physiological differences in the way men and women think or learn), all Texas A & M chemistry students between eighteen and twenty-two (to avoid cultural and age-group differences), all right-handed (to avoid possible differences in right and left hemisphere orientation), all white, monolingual, of average weight and physical activity, non-pregnant, with similar EEG patterns, and in the same stage of their menstrual cycle (the preluteal phase, days five to twelve). He randomly divided the subjects into two groups: a float group and a control group. Both groups underwent a series of seventy-minute learning sessions, during which they listened to taped lessons; all subjects heard identical tapes. The floaters heard the tapes while in the tank; the control group listened while lying relaxed on a sofa in a quiet room that was as dark as the float tank. "The only difference in the two groups was that the experimental group was floating," says Taylor. After the lesson each group was tested (while their brain waves were recorded on the EEG) to determine how much and how well they had learned during the session.

Prompted by his earlier findings that learning takes place on at least three different levels, Taylor tested the subjects on each of those levels. The first, which Taylor calls "basic knowledge," is essentially memorization: How well did the subjects recall the facts they had heard? The second, or "application level," is the ability to understand a concept and use it. The third level, "synthesis thinking," is the ability to put together several concepts and come up with a new idea or an original solution to a problem. A statistical analysis of the results showed that on the first level, floaters did better than the control group. On the second level, the gap between floaters and non-floaters widened. And on the third level, in the extremely complex task of synthesis thought, the superiority of the floating group was greatest of all. "There's no question that the experimental group learned more," said Taylor, "but where they learned is the most important point. People who floated learned at a different cognitive level. The results show that the more difficult the concept, the bigger the difference in the performance of the two groups."

In analyzing the EEG results, Taylor found that floaters produced significantly greater amounts of theta waves. Even more interesting, he discovered that at the moment of comprehending, when all the concepts are brought together in a flash of insight and the problem is suddenly solved (Taylor compares it to a "click" or "mental light bulb going on," and calls it "the Eureka event"), there are sudden changes in the brain waves recorded on the EEG. This moment of synthesis thought, says Taylor, takes place in the theta area. Also significant: He found evidence that visualization helps in learning, and that visualizers did better at all levels of learning.[248]

Lozanov and Superlearning

An extraordinary amount of evidence accumulated in recent years indicates that the greatest amount of learning takes place when the learner's state is one of deep relaxation combined with mental alertness. Perhaps the most influential work has been that of Bulgarian psychiatrist and educator Georgi Lozanov, who has developed a program of accelerated learning he calls "suggestopedia," which involves entering a state of deep relaxation, synchronizing mind and body rhythms through rhythmic breathing, and listening to whatever is to be learned, spoken over a background of slow, rhythmic MUSIC.[148]

Much of Lozanov's work involves the teaching of a foreign language, because language study lends itself to testing: It is quite simple to quantify the new vocabulary presented at each session, and to test the number of words retained at given intervals of months. This type of learning corresponds to what Thomas Taylor called level one, basic knowledge or memorization. The results have been astonishing. While most accelerated-learning or "immersion" language programs consider learning eighty to one hundred words per day extraordinarily successful, and expect a rapid loss of retention, Lozanov's experimental subjects have been able to absorb up to three thousand words per day with the ordinary (i.e., non-experimental) study groups regularly learning up to five hundred words per day. Unlike most accelerated learning programs, which emphasize the necessity of frequent repetition, suggestopedia needs little or no repetition. As for retention, Lozanov's students have virtually total recall after learning, with retention remaining (in one study) at 88 percent six months later. Lozanov's methods and results are now being duplicated at scores of universities and rapid learning institutes in the United States, Canada, and Europe, and applied to learning everything from chemistry to math to poetry. (Lozanov's ideas and techniques are summarized and expanded upon in Sheila Ostrander and Lynn Schroeder's *Superlearning*.[180] This book deals not only with Lozanov, but with other methods of accelerated learning, and includes a wealth of information, including techniques for relaxation, visualization, and suggestions on how to put together tapes for learning. Floaters will find much of the book applicable for in-tank learning programs.)

There are several interdependent explanations for why the Lozanov technique, and other similar superlearning methods, enable people to absorb ideas and information at such an extraordinary rate. First is deep relaxation. As we know, even slight amounts of tension and stress can keep excessive amounts of fight-or-flight biochemicals circulating in the system, and tests have shown that while the fight-or-flight state is fine for executing simple actions, it is not conducive to complex learning. Interestingly, American researchers studying the Lozanov technique have found that not only is deep relaxation essential to the process, but the *deeper the relaxation, the more the student is able to learn.*

One side effect experienced by Lozanov's students was a striking increase in health and general well-being. This can probably be attributed to the stress reduction resulting from frequent long sessions of deep relaxation. And reduction in stress is a crucial factor in learning—a recent test of four thousand children by Georgetown University researchers showed that those who were under emotional or physical stress scored 13 percent lower on I.Q. tests than those who were free of stress.[232]

Also important is the ability to enter the theta state. As Thomas Taylor's study demonstrated, the reverie state of theta is where the mind is most open to the absorption of new material, and in theta the mind is most capable of the complex synthesis thinking—imaginative, visual—that is necessary for combining concepts in new ways, and creating original ideas.

From his emphasis on relaxation, music, and rhythm, it's clear that Lozanov is attempting to involve the right hemisphere in the learning process, since it is the right hemisphere that processes and deals with patterns, rhythms, large-scale and non-detailed material, while the left hemisphere is more effective at detailed, fine-resolution work. Since the left hemisphere is usually dominant, our potential learning capacity is ordinarily crippled; using relaxation and rhythm, Lozanov's technique brings about a cooperation between the hemispheres, with their complementary capacities for processing information. The result is a quantum leap in learning ability.

Another important factor in Lozanov's suggestopedia technique is, as the method's name indicates, the increased suggestibility of the learner. By becoming deeply relaxed and focusing on rhythmic, soothing music, the learner is in a state quite similar to hypnosis, with heightened receptivity to suggestion.

Lozanov also emphasizes the central importance of what he calls de-suggestion—getting rid of a lifetime's accumulation of limiting or negative ideas, such as that we can only learn so much, that we have no aptitude for math or languages, that things like superlearning are impossible. Thus he has his students begin their learning sessions with a series of positive suggestions or affirmations, such as that learning is easy, that the students are calm, confident, capable.

Clearly all the essential elements of the Lozanov technique are present in the float tank experience—and usually to a greater degree:

≈   Relaxation. While Lozanov students often spend several sessions learning how to relax deeply enough to make the method effective, floaters can go rapidly and effortlessly to a state of extremely deep relaxation.

≈   Theta state. The float tank naturally brings about the theta state ideal for the uncritical acceptance of large amounts of new material.

≈   Hemispheric cooperation. Tests show that floating increases access to the right hemisphere and results in a synchronization of the brain-wave activity of the two hemispheres.

≈   Heightened suggestibility. Research indicates that floating leads to a dramatic increase in both suggestibility and the capacity for hypnosis.

≈   De-suggestion. The float tank is a potent tool for what we have discussed earlier as deconditioning, or the unfreezing, changing, and refreezing of belief structures.

In addition to these elements, the float tank has certain characteristics not present in the Lozanov technique, such as the absence of distractions from external stimuli, and the mind's response to sensory deprivation, known as stimulus hunger, which makes the brain even more highly receptive and sensitive to any information presented to it. The float tank is a learning tool of unprecedented power, and while the results of various superlearning programs such as suggestopedia have been remarkable, the float tank has the potential to far surpass them.

Learning in the Tank

The enormous potential of the tank as a tool for enhancing learning ability has been clear to tank manufacturers and researchers for a long time, and there are already a number of superlearning programs in operation that use the tank, playing instruction tapes to floaters through in-tank speakers. So far, these superlearning programs seem to focus mainly on language instruction, using a modified Lozanov technique. However, language learning is mostly a matter of simple memorization, and as Thomas Taylor's study showed, the tank's learning-enhancement effect grows ever stronger as the material to be learned increases in difficulty and complexity. His study concludes that the amplified learning rate that commercial superlearning programs have "reported for the acquisition of a foreign language (a lower cognitive level task) is very small compared to the possible improvement of learning rates for more complex records." [248]

What this means is that we've not even scratched the surface of the tank's promise as an educational tool. Using the tank to learn a language may be rather like using a huge computer to do simple addition. The tank's real power seems to lie in heightening the floater's ability to understand difficult concepts, and to combine these concepts in original and imaginative ways—to come up with new answers to problems, to create new knowledge.

There is no doubt the tank can be a revolutionary instructional tool, with students of all fields of study—biology, economics, music, physics—using the tank as a means of rapidly absorbing large amounts of information and gaining insight into difficult concepts. But where the tank can be of greatest value is on the cutting edge of knowledge—in solving problems, in creating new wisdom and understanding. It's not hard to imagine a nuclear physicist floating, absorbing recent research done by other physicists, reconsidering classical works, and suddenly, in what Thomas Taylor calls a Eureka event, the light clicks on, a new synthesis takes place in his mind, and he has that rarest of blessings: a new idea. Engineers, economists, literary critics, chemists, business executives, lawyers, doctors—all can profit from the augmented capacity for learning, understanding, and thinking that can be gained in the tank. For if the tank's learning-enhancement effect increases as the difficulty and complexity of the material being learned increases, then it must be the scholars, the original thinkers, the finest minds, dealing with the newest and most difficult information and concepts, who will profit most.

Where the real work has yet to be done is in ascertaining how most effectively to present the material to be learned. So far, the most popular method has been to present it verbally, on tape, through in-tank speakers. But researchers are still uncertain about what constitutes the most efficacious presentation on tape. At this point it appears that tape-recorded material is very effective if the information is spoken distinctly, with a certain rhythmic quality, and presented in thought segments, with short pauses between to allow the matter to be digested—which perhaps means to allow it to be transferred from the short-term memory to long-term memory. Following Lozanov, many have found that background music enhances the effect; it should be calming, unobtrusive, beautiful. Ostrander and Schroeder recommend the largo movements of baroque composers, such as Handel, Bach, Vivaldi, Telemann, and Corelli, because they move at a stately rhythm of forty to sixty beats per minute.

Our visual memory is much more powerful than our verbal memory, and many commercial float tanks are now designed to allow the installation of a video screen, so that the floater may satisfy his stimulus hunger by looking upward through the dark to focus with total concentration on a moving image. At least one company, SyberVision, is making videotapes of perfect golf and tennis strokes for "Muscle Memory Programming," using slow motion, different angles, more than one thousand swings, aces, perfect putts, soaring drives, complete with audio sound track of the ball hitting the sweet spot. Described in Chapter Twenty, this kind of visual-motor behavior rehearsal is an enormously useful way to learn and practice, since the body unconsciously absorbs the right moves by a sort of osmosis. But again, this use of visual learning is really only scratching the surface, and present techniques could easily be expanded to include the visual learning of all sports, of dance, painting, and sculpture, how to operate computers or machinery, and much more.

And there's no need to limit visual learning to physical movements. Instruction in mathematics, for example, could combine spoken material with illustrative equations on the video screen, and this combination of eye and ear could be extended to virtually every field of learning. At this point, the only apparent limitation on what and how much can be learned in the tank is our own imagination.

PART FOUR
A NEW PERSPECTIVE
ON FLOATING
(2003)

TWENTY-SIX

THE ENLIGHTENMENT EXPLANATION: FLOATATION AS A GATEWAY TO PURE AWARENESS

One winter's day in 1999 I decided to go for an evening run. Midway through a long run it began to snow heavily and I decided to head for home. On my way home I ran across a foot bridge over the Santa Fe River and halfway across the bridge I slipped on the snow and fell. I bounced once and fell backwards off the bridge down into the rocky riverbed. I hit on the back of my neck against a sharp rock and immediately knew I was paralyzed. My head was out of the water supported by the rock while the rest of my body was submerged in the icy water. I was paralyzed from the neck down and found it hard to breathe so I couldn't call out for help and I couldn't move to try to pull myself out of the river. It was evening and growing dark so I didn't see how anyone would see me in the water. I felt the icy water sucking the heat out of my body and it occurred to me that I was going to die.

I felt an internal ironic chuckle and thought to myself "What a stupid way to go." As the heat drained from my body I began to grow drowsy and recognized the symptoms of hypothermia. At one point I found myself dreaming I was lying in my bed with a river flowing through it and I thought how cold it was and that I should get out of bed but I couldn't seem to move. At the last moments before I passed out I thought: "So this is what it is like to die." I had a feeling that it wasn't bad, in fact it felt very cozy and comfortable, and I realized that after I died I would just pass into this emptiness into which I was already sinking. So I passed out and as far as I knew I died.

The next thing I knew I was waking up on an operating table face-down as a neurosurgeon prepared to surgically fuse my spine. I later found out I had five smashed vertebrae including C2, C3, C5, C6 and T1 and was lucky I was not killed in the fall. Another near death. The surgeon told me I would probably be paralyzed from the neck down for the rest of my life. I was quickly put into a whole upper body cast and head brace that kept my head and neck immobilized with my chin sticking up in the air. The next thing I knew I had a raging case of pneumonia from which the doctors said I almost died. As soon as that pneumonia went away I had another case of pneumonia which was worse than the first. I remember having vivid hallucinations in which I thought I was going to die and that death was an infinite emptiness. There was comfort in that.

As I lay in bed week after week I thought my life was over. I would never walk again, never see my son again, never have sex again, in short I hit rock bottom. Plus I had to wear that damned brace for three months and the inability to move despite my pain was one of the worst experiences I've been through. I thought I've been through four or five near death experiences in just a few days and I tried to figure out if there was some cosmic meaning to that. I remembered the old biblical saying that to be born you must die and I thought that maybe I was unconsciously trying to die so that I could be born again into a new life. But at the time I had no idea what that might mean.

I was determined that I would move again and with much effort, I found I could move my fingers a little bit. I practiced that over and over and it gave me little hope. And then again with much effort I found I could move my foot. Slowly over a period of months I found I could move more and more and I was moved out of intensive care into the hospital rehabilitation ward. There were physical therapists there to help me learn to move more and more of my body. But then because of all the hospital and surgical bills my money ran out and I was forced to be moved out of the hospital into an inexpensive nursing home.

It was a dim, dark, dingy, and depressing old place that was essentially a warehouse for terminal Alzheimer's patients and old people waiting to die. Many of them just lined the hallways sitting all day like vegetables in wheelchairs. Many others were constantly screaming and wandering up-and-down the hallways and sometimes would even wander into my room and climb in bed with me and at times urinate and defecate in my bed. This was frustrating to me since I couldn't move enough to get them out of my bed or room. At first I thought all the constant screaming would drive me crazy. People were dying all the time and often they screamed right up to the time of their death. My roommate kept his TV on from the moment he awoke until the moment he went to sleep. This too was enough to drive me crazy with game shows and talk shows going on all the time.

During the first few months I was seriously depressed. I had never been depressed before and was surprised at how powerful and all-encompassing the experience was—I didn't want to move, I didn't want to get out of bed, I didn't want to think, I was weighted down with an incredible sense of fatigue—as far as I was concerned my life was over. I think at that point I hit rock bottom and if I could have given up and just laid in bed like a vegetable I would have done so. However no matter how depressed I got I never considered suicide. I always had the belief that this accident was some horrible mistake and that somehow I was going to get better. And I always had the feeling that no matter how badly I was damaged I was still me. Because I was still me I often got the feeling that I could just get up and walk although I knew I couldn't move.

I began to think about all my near death experiences and wonder what the meaning of them was. Maybe, I thought, it was a sign that I was gripping onto my life too tightly—that my ego was struggling too hard to be in control—and it was time to let go, let go of my life and let go of my attempts to control my life. The only way I knew to give up the ego was through meditation of which I had some vague knowledge, accumulated over the years. I knew that spiritual masters spoke of becoming enlightened. In some of the books I read it said you didn't have to be religious, worship a God, be the disciple of any particular spiritual master or guru or submit your self to any particular discipline. These books said it was a natural state and that ordinary normal people could become enlightened simply through realizing that they were always already enlightened. Until then I had thought it was only something attained by special, selfless, disciplined, very holy people. I realized that even a non-religious not particularly special person like me could attain enlightenment. I decided that that was the way out of my predicament, and I decided right then and there that I would attain enlightenment.

I had some books on meditation that I had been reading before the accident and I decided the only way to escape the external depressing craziness was to go deep inside myself. The meditation books often talked about having to die—or give up the ego—before you could be born or awakened into enlightenment and I began to think that maybe that was the point of all my near death experiences. Many of the meditation books talked about getting into a state of "no mind" in which you were fully alert and aware but without thoughts, emotions or mind. I would read a few paragraphs of the book and absorb the words, and then close my eyes and try to get into the state of no mind the author was writing about. This involved turning completely inward and ignoring the chaos around me. At first it seemed an impossible task.

But I was determined and practiced from morning until night every day. Soon I found myself having brief periods when there were no thoughts in my mind. Over time these periods lengthened until I found myself spending minutes at a time with no thoughts in my head just existing purely in the present with no thoughts of past or future. As I began to get more and more skilled at getting into a state of no mind I began to realize that it was a feeling I had often had before. The place where I had had that feeling most often was in the floatation tank.

I had floated hundreds of times during the months while I was writing "The Book of Floating" and in the years afterwards when I owned my own tank and spent literally thousands of hours floating. Often while I floated I would get to a state where I was so relaxed my body seemed to dissolve or melt away. At that point I would say to myself "All right, no more words, no more thoughts, no more images, no more mind." Immediately my mind would go blank and I would find myself in a state I could only call "waking dreamless sleep." I was in a state of total blankness and time would disappear. I know I wasn't asleep because I still had a basic primordial awareness even though there were no words or thoughts or images. There was no time because there was no one there to be aware of time—all there was was a blank emptiness that seemed to stretch in all directions infinitely. This blank emptiness seemed to welcome me and there was always a sense that all was well. When I emerged from the blank emptiness in the float tank I always had a sense of enormous well-being, exhilaration and energy. Those floats when I got into the state of total blankness and there was no time were always the best floats of all. When I emerged from the tank I would always be surprised at the time because when I was in the state of blankness there was no time and I could have been there for 10 seconds or two hours. But when I got out of the tank I would be surprised that two or three hours had passed in what seemed like the blink of an eye or a single instant.

Now as I lay in the nursing home reading my books on meditation and going into a state of no mind I realized that what I had been doing in the floatation tank was going into a state of no mind. As I lay in my hospital bed or sat in my wheelchair, I pretended I was in a floatation tank. I shut out all the external noise, closed my eyes, turned my attention completely inward and told myself "no more words, no more thoughts, no more mind". Almost automatically I went into a state of no mind. I was in a state of total silence— all the external screaming and chaos seemed to disappear. I began to spend much of my day in the state of no mind and surprisingly I found I could move more and had more energy and my depression was gone. After about a year of this I was able to get out of bed and walk up-and-down the hallways with a walker. My doctors told me it was a miracle—which is a term doctors don't use very often. My main doctor even took to calling me The Miracle Man.

As I explored the feeling of no mind, or emptiness, I began to discover it had certain qualities. It was infinite in all directions and no matter how deeply into it you went you could always go deeper. It had no inside and no outside—it just "was"—and terms like inside and outside didn't apply because it was everything. It had no center and no edge—of course not, because it was infinite in all directions, it was everything there is. Most importantly this infinite emptiness was totally peaceful—it was ultimate peace and you could stay there forever and never get tired of it, because of course you had no mind to get tired of things and there was no sense of time—it was always just Now with no before and no after.

Then one day something surprising happened. They had come to take me down the hallway in a wheelchair to take a shower. They showered me off and as far as I know I was not in a state of no mind—I was fully involved in taking a shower. Then when they were wheeling me back down the hallway I felt an amazing radiance welling up inside my chest like a spring welling up out of the ground. It seemed to emanate from the center of my chest as if there were a sun inside my chest radiating intensely bright light although there was no light involved—just this powerful invisible radiation welling up. "What is this?" I wondered and by the time I got back to my room I realized that what I was feeling was bliss. I was filled with a sense of excitement and wonder. My life seemed like a miracle.

Sitting there in my wheelchair feeling this extreme bliss I suddenly realized that it wasn't confined to my chest but spread out through my entire body and then throughout the entire room. Everywhere I looked this radiant bliss seem to permeate and interpenetrate everything. In fact it seemed to be like atoms except that it wasn't a material substance—it was invisible like air except it permeated everything including solid objects like it was the secret matrix or substratum of which the entire universe was made. It filled everything and was everywhere and I felt that we humans were like fish swimming in water and wondering "what is this thing called water that everyone talks about?" It was everywhere, all pervasive and so essential and invisible that we couldn't see it and had no idea that it even existed.

I meditated on this and read books looking for similar experiences and decided that what I was perceiving was pure Being, or Consciousness. As I looked around over the next few days seeing this "stuff" that made up everything, it slowly became clear to me that everything was pure Being or Consciousness—everything is Consciousness, Consciousness is all there is, there is only Consciousness. And the blankness and infinite emptiness you go into when you go into the state of no mind is pure Being or Consciousness or primordial Awareness.

As I began more and more to experience Consciousness as everything, my view of life underwent a radical change. I experienced with increasing clarity that if everything is Consciousness, this Consciousness can only be one single unified thing and one thing only. In fact, I realized, Reality is one thing only—Consciousness or pure Being. And if reality is one thing only then ordinary everyday life as we know it is essentially an illusion emerging out of this single unified Being or Reality. This illusion arises out of Consciousness. It's like a movie projected on a screen—we see the actions happening on the screen, tragedy, comedy, drama, and we get involved in the actions and accept the characters as almost real, but in fact they are just projections cast by a single bright light from the projector through the film. The film may run out but the light still shines. That light is Consciousness. It projects everything in the universe and the entire universe is pure illusion. Except of course the metaphor is flawed because Consciousness is everything, even the illusions that it creates or projects to entertain itself.

And since Consciousness is everything and we are all illusions then we are not the doers of our actions. Consciousness lives through us. I began to realize as I walked the hallways of the nursing home that it wasn't me who was doing the walking—Consciousness was walking through me. When I sat in my wheelchair and raised my arm it wasn't me who was raising my arm, it was Consciousness raising my arm. As I realized this, everything became effortless—there was no effort for me to expend since everything I was doing was being done through me by Consciousness. We are not the doers—Consciousness is all there is, there is only Consciousness.

And since there is only Consciousness, and everything that happens is Consciousness, nothing can go wrong. Everything is just the way it is because it is the action of Consciousness. When it comes right down to it we have no choice—all our actions and what we believe to be our decisions are actually the actions of Consciousness. We have no responsibility for what we do or what happens to us—it is all the action of Consciousness. Everything is going to happen just the way it is so why worry about it, just sit back and let it happen because it's going to anyway—there's nothing you can do about it. And when you think you are making choices, that is Consciousness acting through you making you believe that you are making choices when actually it is Consciousness that is acting through you. Seen from this point of view, everything is perfect. Everything is happening perfectly because that is the way Consciousness wants it to happen.

And so I came to the conclusion that everything that had happened to me including my accident and my paralysis was perfect just as it was—it was the result of the actions of Consciousness moving through my life. The facts that I had no choice and that everything was perfect just the way it was was a tremendous relief to me and lifted from me a great burden of responsibility and regret.

After two years in the nursing home and over a year of almost constant meditation I was able to walk well enough to be released from the nursing home and go to live in my own apartment which was provided for me by public housing. There I continued meditating and the feeling of bliss continued to well up inside me. My hands were still paralyzed and the rest of my body was still partially paralyzed. So people were paid by the state to come by for a few hours in the morning to get me out of bed and get dressed and make me breakfast, then someone came by later in the evening to make me dinner and get me into bed. All the rest of the day I'm blissfully by myself and I spend much of my time in a state of no mind. I have joined a gym, and my helper takes me out and helps me get onto the Nautilus machines and pump iron. I have come a long way from when the doctors were telling me I would never move again from the neck down. I am living in poverty but it is blissful poverty. And I realize that everything is perfect just the way it is.

As soon as I was able I made a trip down to Albuquerque to a float center where I took a float. As I got into the tank the voice in my head said, "ah, home again!" As I relaxed back into the tank I felt all the contractions—contractions of the body, of the emotions and of the mind—release and let go completely and my body dissolved into delicious and blissful state of comfort and peace. This is one thing I had forgotten about floating. All my meditation had been done lying in bed or sitting in my wheelchair. There, no matter how relaxed you get you still feel the pressure of the bed or the chair against the back of your body. Now, back in the tank again I floated freely on top of the Epsom salts solution and it was as if gravity had disappeared and I was floating in space with no pressure against my back or any part of my body. I was able to let go completely of all contractions and all sense of pressure. After a few minutes of releasing all contractions and tensions, my body had let go completely and dissolved into pure relaxation.

I said to myself what I usually had said whenever I floated before the accident. I said "No more words, no more thoughts, no more images, no more mind." Almost immediately all words in my head ceased, there were no more thoughts, since thoughts require words, all images disappeared into the vast infinite emptiness, and I found myself in the state of no mind.

As I had suspected it would be, It was the same state I had discovered in my meditations in the long years in the nursing home. No mind is no mind no matter where it happens but it was clear that the floatation tank facilitated the process and speeded it up enormously.

As I lay there in timeless pure Being, black empty space extended infinitely in all directions and my body ceased to exist. It was clear to me that everything was Consciousness—pure primordial Consciousness with no content whatsoever, just emptiness and silence and total stillness. How could anything move because it was pure emptiness and was a totally solid field which was everything. There was no more me, I had disappeared, and all that was left was what is eternally present and never changes.

It became clear to me that I had been in this state hundreds of times in the decade and a half before the accident when I had been in the floatation tank. But because I had read no spiritual literature and had no experience with spiritual reality I had no idea that that was what was happening to me. I simply assumed that I had become so relaxed in the tank that I went into a blank state on the verge of sleep where I had no thoughts and no memories and no sense of time. It just seemed to be a normal part of what I would call a "good float." It didn't happen every float but when it did I always emerged from the tank with an extraordinary sense of being deeply rested and filled with energy and exhilaration.

After the floats when I went into the state of no mind as I went out into the world my senses were extremely—almost unbelievably—sharp and keen. Everything I saw seemed beautiful and miraculous and the colors of everything were extraordinarily rich and beautiful. I saw everything clearly as if objects had sharp edges around them. It was as if you normally have to wear glasses because without them everything is fuzzy, and then you put on your glasses and suddenly everything comes into sharp clarity. But I didn't wear glasses and everything became much more sharp and clear than it normally was. My sense of smell was fantastically keen and walking through the streets became an exhilarating experience of being bombarded by hundreds of different smells. I could smell the perfume on women as much as a block away and the smell of trees and flowers was rich and delightful. My sense of hearing had increased sharply and as I walked through the streets I could overhear and listen fully to scores of different conversations at the same time, some of them as far as a block away. Everything seemed delightful and I had a powerful sense that all was well. The world itself seemed miraculous and I was totally and intensely in the present moment without thinking of past or future. Everything I did seemed to come effortlessly and easily.

At the time I just assumed that this was the result of a good float. But now in the years since my accident I have read many spiritual books, done much meditation, spoken with many spiritual masters, and have had what you might call an experience of awakening, and it has become clear to me that this sense of awakening is not the necessary or inevitable result of floating, but the result of something that can happen to you while you are floating. The float tank is like a gateway to infinite being. It doesn't necessarily put you into a state of no mind or make you aware of pure Being, or open your eyes to the fact that Consciousness is all there is, that everything is Consciousness, that there is only Consciousness. These realizations come from the repeated experience of no mind and learning to abide in no mind or pure Being for long periods of time. Experiences in the float tank makes this possible and the float tank is the most effective tool I am aware of for having these experiences.

Ordinarily this takes an enormous amount of practice. You must learn to abide intensely in the present moment with no before and no after. Thoughts arise but if you apply yourself to discovering the source of your thoughts you find they arise out of emptiness, pure Consciousness without content. In ordinary life this usually takes a relatively long period of practice. But the float tank is an ideal tool for accelerating the process. It is a perfect environment for releasing all contractions, letting go of the distractions of the body and mind, and becoming so profoundly relaxed that it becomes easier to let go of all thoughts, emotions, images, and the mind itself and abide in a state of no mind.

It's wonderful to be able to go quickly into a state of no mind, for which the floatation tank is an ideal tool. However unless you have a sense of the spiritual reality to which no mind is the doorway, you may miss the experience completely and think you've just had a momentary lapse of Consciousness or brief period of blankness or sleep. My recommendation is that in addition to floating you do some reading of spiritual literature that will give you a context for the experiences you are having in the tank. In fact reading spiritual literature will speed up and facilitate the process of spiritual awakening in the tank.

Let me briefly mention a few of the books that were particularly helpful during my years in the nursing home in teaching me to enter a state of no mind. One powerful little book is *The Power of Now: A Guide to Spiritual Enlightenment*, by Eckhart Tolle. This book is a clear and straightforward description of how to live fully in the Now, and shows you how you can enter pure Being through feeling the inner body and passing through the inner body into the infinite emptiness of primordial awareness. *I Am That*, a series of dialogues with the Indian sage Sri Nisargadatta is an endless series of awakening lessons by a fully enlightened master. The books *The Open Secret* and *As It Is* by the British teacher Tony Parsons present a series of exceptional dialogues and essays that emphasize the pure simplicity of waking Consciousness, which is eternally present and constitutes all there is. The dialogues of Ramana Maharshi, who is surely the greatest sage of recent centuries, are astonishing in their clarity and their insistence that we are always already enlightened; we just need to become aware of it. I recommend the recently published *Talks with Ramana Maharshi*. His words carry a special power and charisma that are able to put you immediately into a state of no mind. Some of the books of Poonjaji, also known as Papaji, such as *Wake Up and Roar* are dialogues from a completely awakened man that have the power to awaken the reader.

Papaji was for many years a disciple of Ramana Maharshi. Then beginning in the late 80s many Westerners went to India to study with Papaji and he had the power to bring hundreds of them into a state of awakening. These disciples of Papaji are now in the West writing their own books and traveling from town to town giving talks and meditations. Perhaps the most well-known of Papaji's disciples is a woman named Gangaji, who has written several powerful books and travels the world giving talks and meditations.

I also gained much insight from reading Zen literature, for the Zen experience of Satori or Kensho is exactly the same as waking up to the experience of no mind and the realization that everything is Consciousness. I particularly recommend some of the ancient Zen masters such as Bankei, Dogen and many others. They spent many hours in meditation cutting off all thoughts and I can't help but think that their experiences in solitude have much in common with spending time in the floatation tank. Solitude, I believe, is definitely a necessity for entering a state of no mind.

I remember that when I was in my early 20s I spent several years living in isolation and solitude in a crude lean-to way up the side of the mountain in the wilderness miles from the nearest road. There was no electricity or running water of course, and I took my drinking water out of the stream that ran past my lean-to. I would often go for weeks at a time without speaking to anyone or seeing anyone. After several months I noticed that my mind would often go completely blank and I seemed to be existing in a timeless state. When the winter came the mountains and trees were covered with snow and the sky would be a whitish shade of gray so that I was totally surrounded by whiteness. This increased the feeling of sensory deprivation. My senses became extremely sharp and I noticed that for long periods my mind was a total blank and I lost all sense of time—there was no time. I was in a state of absolute peace. I felt I was on the verge of discovering something important.

A friend of mine had given me a book by John Lilly about the floatation tank. As I read it I became more and more amazed because the experiences that John Lilly described having in the floatation tank were in many ways identical to the experiences I was having in my own state of sensory deprivation on the mountainside. I immediately wanted to go out and find a floatation tank. I vowed that as soon as I could find a floatation tank I would have the experience. Because it seemed like John Lilly was able to have the same experiences in the float tank in just a few minutes that it had taken me months to achieve in my mountaintop isolation.

In the end it took me over ten years before I got a magazine assignment to write about the floatation tank and I began floating regularly in the float center near my apartment in New York City. Out of that magazine article, with the addition of about a year of scientific research, emerged *The Book of Floating*. The book had chapters based on scientific evidence about the various psychobiological changes and experiences that happened in the float tank. But it had no chapter on the spiritual aspects of floating, simply because I wasn't aware of them. With all my experiences of timelessness and periods of no thoughts you would have thought I might have become aware that I was going through spiritual experiences. But to me they were just blank periods and I didn't consider them anything special. In fact they are absolutely not special—they are just the emergence of primordial awareness and emptiness which is eternally present and is the substratum of all existence—it never comes and never goes, is never born and never dies, is one solid Reality which is everything that exists. It is always there and once you become aware of it you realize it has always been present in your life and is nothing extraordinary.

It wasn't until I had my near death experiences and realized that this Reality which was present in life continued to be present in death, that I began to get the feeling that this was pure Being and was eternally present. In the nursing home as I meditated until I could get myself into a state of no mind I finally began to realize that this was the spiritual experience written about by the sages and spiritual masters. That was the point when I understood that this experience was nothing new to me but that I had been into it hundreds of times during my periods of "wakeful deep sleep" or Consciousness with no content in the floatation tank.

It can happen naturally in the float tank if you allow yourself to sink into deep relaxation. First you let go of all contractions and constrictions and let your body seem to dissolve until you reach what seems like the bottom of all relaxation—the deepest you can go. Then if you rest there a while you'll find that you can relax even more as if all your body is melting away. Then you continue going deeper and come to rest at the ultimate state of relaxation. At that point you may find your thoughts and feelings and emotions disappearing. If you let that happen fully and give up all resistance you may find yourself sinking into a state of no mind. For me the quickest way is after I have reached the state of deepest relaxation I simply say to myself in my mind, "no more words, no more thoughts, no more images, no more mind." Amazingly as soon as I say this to myself my mind becomes empty of words thoughts and images and I am in the blankness of no mind where there is no time because it is always exactly that moment that never changes and has no before and no after.

—Michael Hutchison
mhutchisonmn@aol.com

BIBLIOGRAPHY

(The numbers preceding these entries correspond to the reference numbers given within the text of the book; e.g., number 170, John Naisbitt's *Megatrends*, is referred to on page 34.)

1. Adam, J. E. "Naloxone Reversal of Analgesia Produced by Brain Stimulation in the Human." *Pain*, Vol. 2 (1976), pp. 161-166.

2. Ader, R., ed. *Psychoneuroimmunology*. New York: Academic Press, 1981.

3. Agras, W. S., M. Horne and C. B. Taylor. "Expectations and the Blood-Pressure-Lowering Effects of Relaxation." *Psychosomatic Medicine*, Vol. 44 (1982), pp. 389-395.

4. Applewhite Philip B., *Molecular Gods: How Molecules Determine Our Behavior.* Englewood Cliffs, N.J.: Prentice-Hall, 1981.

5. Assagioli, Roberto. *Psychosynthesis.* New York: Viking Press. 1971.

6. ————. *The Act of Will.* New York: Viking Press, 1973.

7. Azima, H., and F. J. Cramer "Effects of Decrease in Sensory Variability on Body Scheme." *Canadian Journal of Psychiatry*, Vol. I (1956), pp. 59-72.

8. Bailey, Ronald H. et al. *The Role of the Brain.* New York: Time-Life Books, 1975.

9. Baltimore, David. "Psychology Tomorrow: The Nobel View." *Psychology Today* (December 1982).

10. Banquet, J. P. "EEG and Meditation." *Journal of Electroencephalography and Clinical Neurophysiology*, Vol. 33 (1972), pp. 449-458

11. ————. "Spectral Analysis of EEG and Meditation." *Journal of Electroencephalography and Clinical Neurophysiology*. Vol 35 (1973). pp. 143-151.

12. Barabasz, Arreed E. "Effects of Brief and Long Term REST on Conformity of Perception of Figure Inversion." Paper delivered at First International Conference on REST and Self-Regulation, Denver, Colorado, March 17, 1983.

13. ———. "Restricted Environmental Stimulation and the Enhancement of Hypnotizability: Pain, EEC, Alpha. Skin Conductance and Temperature Responses." *The International Journal of Clinical and Experimental Hypnosis*, Vol. 2 (1982), pp. 147-166.

14. Barfield, A. "Biological Influences on Sex Differences in Behavior." in Michael S. Teitelbaum, *Sex Differences*. Garden City, N.Y.: Anchor Press, 1976.

15. Basmajian, John V. *Muscles Alive: Their Functions Revealed by Electromyography*. Baltimore: Williams & Wilkins, 1962.

16. ———. "Control and training of individual motor units." *Science*, Vol. 141 (1963), pp: 440-441.

17. ———, ed. *Biofeedback—Principles and Practice for Clinicians*. Baltimore: Wilhams & Wilkins, 1979

18. Beisser, A. R. "Denial and Affirmation in Illness and Health." *American Journal of Psychiatry*, Vol. 136 (1979), 1,026-1,030.

19. Belden, Allen, and Gregg Jacobs. "REST in a Hospital-Based Stress Management Program." Paper delivered at First International Conference on REST and Self-Regulation, Denver, Colorado, March 17, 1983.

20. Belson, Abby Avin. "New Focus on Chemistry of Joylessness." *The New York Times* (March 15, 1983).

21. Benson, Herbert. *The Relaxation Response*. New York: William Morrow, 1975.

22. ———. *The Mind/Body Effect: How Behavioral Medicine Can Show You the Way to Better Health*. New York: Simon & Schuster, 1979.

23. ———, et al. "Historical and Clinical Considerations of the Relaxation Response." *American Scientist* (July-August 1977):

24. ———, and R. K. Wallace. "Decreased Drug Abuse with Transcendental Meditation: A Study of 1,862 Subjects." *Congressional Record*, 92nd Congress, 1st Session, June 1971.

25. Bentov, Itzhak. *Stalking the Wild Pendulum: On the Mechanics of Consciousness*. New York: E. P. Dutton, 1977.

26. Bernhardt, Dr. Roger, and David Martin: *Self-Mastery Through Self-Hypnosis*. Indianapolis: Bobbs-Merrill, 1977:

27. Bexton, W. H., W. Heron, and T. H. Scott. Effects of Decreased Variation in the Sensory Environment. *Canadian Journal of Psychology*, Vol. 8 (1954), pp. 70-76.

28. Black, David: "Lie Down in Darkness." *New York* magazine (December 10, 1979).

29. Blackwell, B. "The Endorphins: Current Psychiatric Research." *Psychiatric Opinion* (October 1979).

30. Blakeslee, Thomas R. *The Right Brain*. New York: Doubleday, 1980

31. Borrie, Roderick A., and Peter Suedfeld. "Restricted Environmental Stimulation Therapy in a Weight Reduction Program." *Journal of Behavioral Medicine*, Vol. 3 (1980), pp: 147-161.

32. "The Brain." *Scientific American* (September 1979), entire issue.

33. Brockmeyer, Arthur: "Floating and Asthma Reduction: A Case Study and Baseline Study Formula." Paper delivered at First International Conference on REST and Self-Regulation, Denver, Colorado, March 17, 1983.

34. Brody, Jane E: "Emotions Found to Influence Nearly Every Human Ailment." *The New York Times* (May 24, 1983).

35. Bross, Michael. "The Application of Sensory Restriction Techniques in the Study of Sensory Functions." Paper delivered at First International Conference on REST and Self-Regulation, Denver, Colorado, March 17, 1983.

36. Budiansky, Stephen. "Pain." *SciQuest* (December 1981).

37. Budzynski, Thomas: "Tuning In on the Twilight Zone." *Psychology Today* (August 1977).

38. ———. "A Brain Lateralization Model for REST." Paper delivered at First International Conference on REST and Self-Regulation, Denver Colorado, March 18, 1983.

39. ———, and K. Peffer. "Twilight state learning: The presentation of learning material during a biofeedback-produced altered state." Denver: Biofeedback Research Society, 1974

40. Cade, C. Maxwell, and Nona Coxhead. *The Awakened Mind: Biofeedback and the Development of Higher States of Awareness*. New York: Delacorte Press, 1979.

41. Cahn, Harold. "A Novel Application of Sensory Isolation: Tank Training to Reduce Sickness Absenteeism in City of Phoenix Employees." Paper delivered at First International Conference on REST and Self-Regulation, Denver Colorado, March 17, 1983.

42. Calvin, William H., Ph.D., and George A. Ojemann, M.D. *Inside the Brain: Mapping the Cortex, Exploring the Neuron.* New York: New American Library, 1980.

43. "Canadian study frames new right/left paradigm." *Brain/Mind Bulletin,* Vol. 8 (March 28, 1983) p.7

44. Cannon, Walter B. *The Wisdom of the Body,* New York: W: W. Norton, 1932.

45. Carrington, Patricia, Ph.D. *Freedom in Meditation.* New York: Anchor Press, Doubleday, 1978.

46. Collins, Glenn. "A New Look at Anxiety's Many Faces." *The New York Times* (January 24, 1983).

47. ———, "Chemical Connections: Pathways of Love." *The New York Times* (February 14, 1983).

48. Cooper. L., and Milton Erickson. *Time Distortion in Hypnosis.* Baltimore: William and Wilkins, 1954.

49. Cousins, Norman: "Anatomy of an Illness (as Perceived by the Patient):" *New England Journal of Medicine,* Vol. 295 (1976), pp. 1.458-1,463.

50. ———. "Potentiation and the Patient." Bulletin of the American College of Surgeons (June 1980).

51. ———. *The Healing Heart: Antidotes to Panic and Helplessness.* New York. W. W. Norton, 1983.

52. Csikszentmihalyi, Mihaly. *Beyond Boredom and Anxiety: The Experience of Play in Work and Games.* San Francisco and London: Jossey-Bass, 1975.

53. Daniel, Alma: "Uses of REST in a Private Practice Utilizing a Flotation Tank:" Paper delivered at First International Conference on REST and Self-Regulation, Denver, Colorado, March 17, 1983.

54. Darden, Ellington. *The Athlete's Guide to Sports Medicine.* Chicago: Contemporary Books, 1981.

55. ———. *The Nautilus Bodybuilding Book.* Chicago: Contemporary Books, 1982.

56. Deikman, A. J. "Deautomatization and the Mystic Experience:" *Psychiatry,* Vol. 29 (1966)s pp: 324-338.

57. "Experimental Meditation." *Journal of Nervous and Mental Disorders*, Vol. 136 (1963), pp. 329-373.

58. "Depressed Lymphocytes." *Science News*, Vol. 121 (1983), P. 360.

59. Dent, Jim. "Mental Conditioning Boosts Septien's Boots." *Dallas Times Herald* (September 18, 1981).

60. DiCara, Leo. "Learning in the Autonomic Nervous System." *Scientific American* (January 1970).

61. ————, ed. *Recent Advances in Limbic and Autonomous Nervous System Research*. New York: Plenum, 1973.

62. Dossey, Larry, M.D. *Space, Time & Medicine*. Boulder, Col.: Shambhala, 1982.

63. Driscoll, R. "Anxiety Reduction Using Physical Exertion and Positive Images." *Physiological Record*, Vol. 26 (1976), pp. 87-94.

64. Eccles, John C. *The Understanding of the Brain*. New York: McGraw-Hill, 1977.

65. Eliade, Mircea. *Yoga: Immortality and Freedom*. Princeton, N.J.: Princeton University Press. 1969.

66. "Endorphin link to pain relief is confirmed." *Medical World News* (February 19, 1979).

67. "The Endorphins – The Body's Own Opiates." *The Harvard Medical School Health Letter* (January 1983).

68. "Evidence sheds new light on prior right/left assumptions." *Brain/Mind Bulletin*, Vol. 8 (March 28, 1983), p. 7.

69. Feldenkrais, Moshe. *Awareness Through Movement: Health Exercises for Personal Growth*. New York: Harper & Row, 1972.

70. ————. *Body and Mature Behavior: A Study of Anxiety, Sex, Gravitation and Learning*. New York: International Universities Press, 1970.

71. Ferguson, Marilyn. *The Brain Revolution*. New York: Bantam Books, 1975. ————

72. Fields, H. L. "Secrets of the Placebo." *Psychology Today* (November 1978).

73. Fine, Thomas H. "REST in the Treatment of Essential Hypertension." Paper delivered at First International Conference on REST and Self-Regulation, Denver, Colorado, March 17, 1983.

74. ————, and John W. Turner, Jr. "Restricted Environmental Stimulation Therapy: A New Relaxation Model." Unpublished paper.

75. French, J. D. "The Reticular Formation." *Physiological Psychology: Readings from Scientific American.* San Francisco: W. H. Freeman, 1975.

76. Friedman, Meyer, and Ray H. Rosenman. *Type A Behavior and Your Heart.* New York: Alfred A. Knopf, 1974.

77. Friedman, R C., et al. *Sex Differences in Behavior.* New York: John Wiley & Sons, 1974.

78. Gallwey, W. Timothy. *The Inner Game of Tennis.* New York: Random House, 1974.

79. ⸺⸺, *Inner Tennis: Playing the Game.* New York: Random House, 1976.

80. Gatchel, Robert J., and Kenneth P. Price, eds. *Clinical Applications of Biofeedback: Appraisal & Status.* New York: Pergamon Press, 1979.

81. Gazzaniga, M. S. *The Bisected Brain.* New York: Appleton-Century-Crofts, 1974.

82. ⸺⸺, and J. E. LeDoux. *The Integrated Mind.* New York: Plenum, 1978.

83. Glasser, William. *Positive Addiction.* New York: Harper & Row, 1976.

84. Glueck, Bernard C., and C. F. Stroebel. "Biofeedback and Meditation in the Treatment of Psychiatric Illness." *Comprehensive Psychiatry,* Vol. 16 (1975), pp. 303-321.

85. Grant, Mark. "'Tranquillity Tank': Rehab Fad or Fact?" *Medical News* (November 2, 1981).

86. "The Great Tank Escape." *Newsweek* (May 4, 1981).

87. Green, Elmer, and Alyce Green. *Beyond Biofeedback.* New York: Delacorte Press, 1977.

88. Gregg, Sandra R. "Psychologist Floats a New Concept for Reducing Stress in Patients." *The Washington Post* (December 26, 1982).

89. Guillemin, Roger. "Peptides in the Brain: The New Endocrinology of the Neurone." *Science* Vol. 202 (1978), pp. 390-402.

90. ⸺⸺, and Roger Burgus. "The Hormones of the Hypothalamus." *Scientific American* (November 1972).

91. Haber, Ralph. "How We Remember What We See." *Scientific American* (May 1970).

92. Hales, Dianne. "Psycho-Immunity." *Science Digest* (November 1981).

93. Halpern, Howard. *How to Break Your Addiction to a Person.* New York: McGraw-Hill, 1982.

94. Hampden-Turner, Charles. *Maps of the Mind.* New York: Macmillan, 1981.

95. Harris, A. "Sensory Deprivation and Schizophrenia." *Journal of Mental Science,* Vol. 105 (1959), pp. 235-237.

96. Harris, Roy J., Jr. "In the Darkest Dark of the 'Lilly Pond' Floats Our Reporter." *The Wall Street Journal* (May 8, 1980).

97. Hatterer, Dr. Lawrence J. *The Pleasure Addicts.* Cranbury, N.J.: A. S. Barnes, 1980.

98. Henry, James P. "Present Concept of Stress Theory," in *Catecholamines and Stress: Recent Advances,* eds. Earl Usdin, Richard Kvetriansky, and Irwin Kopin. *Developments in Neuroscience.* Volume 8. New York, Amsterdam, and Oxford: Elsevier North-Holland, 1980.

99. Heron, Woodburn. "The Pathology of Boredom." *Scientific American* (January 1957).

100. Higdon, Hal. "Loosen Up and Fly Right." *The Runner* (May 1983).

101. Hooper, Judith. "Releasing the Mystic in Your Brain." *Science Digest* (May 1981).

102. ──────. "Interview with Candace Pert," *Omni* (February 1982).

103. "Hormones Tied to Heart Ills." *The New York Times* (October 24, 1982).

104. "How the Brain Works." *Newsweek* (February 7, 1983).

105. Hughes. J., et al. "Identification of two related pentapeptides from the brain with potent opiate antagonist activity." *Nature,* Vol. 258 (1975), pp. 577-579.

106. Hunt, Roy Arthur. "Naming an Unknown World: The Transformation of Perceived Meaning by Voluntary Subjects After Repeated Use of the 'Isolation Tank' Flotation Environment." Unpublished dissertation, Boston University, 1980.

107. Hutchison, Mike. "Isolation Tanks: The State of the Art." *Esquire* (August 1983).

108. ──────. "Tanks for the Memories," *The Village Voice* (July 13, 1982).

109. ──────. "The Syncro-Energizer: Letting a Black Box Meditate for You," *Esquire* (February 1984).

110. Iverson, Leslie L. "The Chemistry of the Brain." *Scientific American* (September 1979).

111. Jacobs, Gregg, Robert Heilbronner, and John M. Stanley. "The Effects of Short-Term Flotation REST on Relaxation: A Controlled Study," Paper delivered at First International Conference on REST and Self-Regulation, Denver, Colorado, March 18, 1983.

112. ————. "The Effects of Sensory Isolation on Relaxation," Unpublished paper.

113. Jacobson, Edmund, M.D. "Imagination of Movement Involving Skeletal Muscle." *American Journal of Physiology*, Vol. 91 (1930), pp, 567-608.

114. ————. "Evidence of Contraction of Specific Muscles during Imagination," *American Journal of Physiology*, Vol. 9.5 (1930), pp, 703-712.

115. ————. *Progressive Relaxation*, revised. Chicago: University of Chicago Press, 1938.

116. ————. *You Must Relax*, rev. ed. New York, Toronto, and London: McGraw-Hill, 1962.

117. Jaffe, Dennis T., Ph.D. *Healing from Within*. New York: Alfred A. Knopf, 1980.

118. Janda, Louis. "REST in the Treatment of Obesity." Paper delivered at First International Conference on REST and Self-Regulation, Denver, Colorado, March 17, 1983.

119. Jaynes, Julian, *The Origins of Consciousness in the Breakdown of the Bicameral Mind*. Boston: Houghton Mifflin, 1976.

120. Jevning, R. "Meditation increased blood flow to brain in UC study." *Brain/Mind Bulletin*, Vol. 4 (January 15, 1979), p. 1.

121. Jonas, Gerald. *Visceral Learning*. New York: Viking Press, 1973.

122. Jung, C. G. *Memories, Dreams, Reflections*. New York: Pantheon Books, 1963.

123. ————. *The Portable Jung*, ed. Joseph Campbell. New York: Viking Press, 1971.

124. ————, et al. *Man and His Symbols*. Garden City, N.Y.: Doubleday, 1964.

125. Kammerman, M., ed. *Sensory Isolation and Personality Change*, Springfield, Ill.: Charles C, Thomas, 1977.

126. Karlins, Marvin, and Lewis M. Andrews. *Bio-Feedback*. New York: Warner Books, 1972.

127. Kasamatsu, A., and T. Hirai. "Science of Zazen." *Psychologia*, Vol. 6 (1963), pp. 86-91.

128. "The Keys to Paradise." *Nova: Adventures in Science*. Boston: Addison-Wesley, 1982.

129. Kinsbourne, Marcel. "Sad Hemisphere, Happy Hemisphere," *Psychology Today* (May 1981).

130. Koestler, Arthur. *The Act of Creation*. New York: Macmillan, 1964.

131. ———. *The Ghost in the Machine*. New York: Random House. 1967.

132. Kostrubala, Thaddeus. *The Joy of Running*. Philadelphia: Lippincott, 1976.

133. LeCron, Leslie M. *Self Hypnotism*. Englewood Cliffs, N.J.: Prentice-Hall, 1964.

134. Lenard, Lane. "Visions that Vanquish Cancer." *Science Digest* (April 1981).

135. J. Leonard, George. *The Ultimate Athlete*. New York: Viking Press, 1975.

136. ———. *The Silent Puls*. New York: E. P. Dutton, 1978.

137. Levine, J. B., et al. "The Narcotic Antagonist Naloxone Enhances Clinical Pain," *Nature*, Vol. 272 (1978), pp. 826-827.

138. Lilly, John C., M.D. *The Center of the Cyclone*, New York: Julian press, 1972.

139. ———. *The Deep Self*. New York: Simon & Schuster, 1977.

140. ———. *The Scientist*. New York: J. B. Lippincott, 1978.

141. ———. "Interview." *Omni* (January 1983).

142. ———. and Jay T. Shurley. "Experiments in Solitude, in Maximum Achievable Physical Isolation with Water Suspension, of Intact Healthy Persons," in *Psychophysiological Aspects of Space Flight*, ed. B. E. Flaherty. New York: Columbia University Press, 1961.

143. Lord, J. A. H., et al. "Endogenous Opioid Peptides: Multiple Agonists and Receptors," *Nature*, Vol. 267 (1977), pp. 495-499.

144. Lowen, Alexander, M.D. *The Betrayal of the Body*, New York: Collier, 1969.

145. ———. *Pleasure: A Creative Approach to Life*. New York: Coward, McCann & Geoghegan, 1970.

146. ———. *Depression and the Body: The Biological Basis of Faith and Reality*, New York: Coward, McCann & Geoghegan, 1972.

147. "Lowering Blood Pressure without Drugs" (editorial), *Lancet* (August 30, 1980).

148. Lozanov, Georgi. *Suggestology and Outlines of Suggestopedy.* New York: Gordon & Breach, 1982.

149. Lynch, Dudley. "Creative Flashes from the Twilight Zone." *Science Digest* (December 1981).

150. McAuliffe, Kathleen, "Brain Tuner." *Omni* (January 1983).

151. Maccoby, Eleanor E. *The Development of Sex Differences.* Palo Alto, Cal.: Stanford University Press, 1966.

152. McGaugh, J. L., ed. *The Chemistry of Mood, Motivation and Memory.* New York: Plenum, 1972.

153. MacLean, Paul D, "Contrasting Functions of Limbic and Neocortical Systems of the Brain and their Relevance to Psycho-physiological Aspects of Medicine." *American Journal of Medicine,* Vol. 25 (1958), pp. 611-626.

154. ———. "New Findings Relevant to the Evolution of Psychosexual Functions of the Brain." *Journal of Nervous and Mental Disease,* Vol. 13.5 (1962), pp, 289-296.

155. ———. "The Paranoid Streak in Man." in *Beyond Reductionism,* eds. Arthur Koestler and J. R. Smythies. Boston: Beacon Press, 1969.

156. ———. *A Triune Concept of the Brain and Behavior.* Toronto: University of Toronto Press, 1973.

157. Maier, W. J. "Sensory Deprivation Therapy of an Autistic Boy." *American Journal of Psychotherapy,* Vol. 25 (1970), pp. 228-245.

158. Maslow, Abraham. *Motivation and Personality.* New York: Harper & Brothers, 1954.

159. ———. *Towards a Psychology of Being.* Princeton, N.J.: Van Nostrand, 1962.

160. ———. *Religions, Values, and Peak Experiences.* New York: Viking Press, 1970.

161. ———. *The Farther Reaches of Human Nature.* New York: Viking Press, 1971.

162. Matthews-Simonton, Stephanie. "Visualization and Healing." Speech delivered to Symposium on Healing in Our Time, Washington, D.C., October 21, 1982.

163. Mayer, D. J., D. D. Price, and A. Raffil. "Antagonism of acupuncture analgesia in man by the narcotic antagonist naloxone." *Brain Research*, Vol. 121 (1977), pp. 360-373.

164. Meredith, Dennis. "Healing with Electricity." *Science Digest* (May 1981).

165. Miele, Philip. "The Power of Suggestion: A New Way of Learning Languages." *Parade* (March 12, 1978).

166. Miller, Jonathan. *States of Mind.* New York: Pantheon Books, 1983.

167. Miller, N., and L. DiCara. "Instrumental learning of urine formation by rats; changes in renal blood flow." *American Journal of Physiology*, Vol. 215 (1968), pp. 677-683.

168. Morgan, Elaine. *The Aquatic Ape: A Theory of Human Evolution.* New York: Stein & Day, 1982.

169. Mutke, Peter H. C., M.D. *Selective Awareness.* Millbrae, Cal.: Celestial Arts, 1976.

170. Naisbitt, John. *Megatrends: Ten New Directions Transforming Our Lives.* New York: Warner Books, 1982.

171. Naranjo, Claudio, and Robert E. Ornstein. *On the Psychology of Meditation.* New York: Viking Press, 1971.

172. Nicklaus, Jack, with Ken Bowden. *Golf My Way.* New York: Simon & Schuster, 1974.

173. Nuernberger, Phil, Ph.D. *Freedom from Stress: A Holistic Approach.* Honesdale, Pa.: Himalayan Institute, 1981.

174. Olds, J. "Pleasure Centers in the Brain." *Scientific American*, Vol. 195 (1956), pp. 105-116.

175. ————. "The Central Nervous System and the Reinforcement of Behavior." *American Psychologist*, Vol. 24 (1969), pp. 707-719.

176. O'Leary, Daniel S., and Robert L. Heilbronner. "Flotation REST and Information Processing: A Reaction-Time Study." Paper delivered at First International Conference on REST and Self-Regulation, Denver, Colorado, March 17, 1983.

177. Ornstein, Robert E. *On the Experience of Time.* New York: Penguin Books, 1969.

178. ————. *The Psychology of Consciousness.* San Francisco: W. H. Freeman, 1972.

179. ————. ed. *The Nature of Human Consciousness.* New York: Viking Press, 1974.

180. Ostrander, Sheila, and Lyn Schroeder, with Nancy Ostrander. *Superlearning.* New York: Delacorte Press, 1979.

181. Oyle, Irving, M.D. *The New American Medicine Show: Discovering the Healing Connection.* Santa Cruz, Cal.: Unity Press, 1979.

182. ————. *The Healing Mind.* Millbrae, Cal.: Celestial Arts, 1979.

183. Paasch, Hope. "Wet behind the ears, but learning fast: study shows floating good for students." *The Texas A & M Battalion* (August 12, 1982).

184. "Pain: Placebo Effect Linked to Endorphins" *Science News* (September 2, 1978).

185. Patel, Chandra. "Reduction of Serum Cholesterol and Blood Pressure in Hypertensive Patients by Behavior Modification." *Journal of the Royal College of General Practitioners,* Vol. 26 (1976), P. 111.

186. Pelletier, Kenneth R. *Mind as Healer, Mind as Slayer.* New York: Delacorte Press, 1977.

187. ————. *Toward a Science of Consciousness.* New York: Delacorte Press, 1978.

188. ————. *Longevity.* New York: Delacorte Press, 1981.

189. Perry, Glenn A., and Lee Perry. "A Discussion of the Use of the Floatation Tank in Public Settings for Commercial Uses." Paper delivered at First International Conference on REST and Self-Regulation, Denver, Colorado, March 17, 1983.

190. Pert, Candace. "Interview." *Omni* (February 1982).

191. *Physiological Psychology: Readings from Scientific American.* San Francisco: W. H. Freeman. 1971.

192. Pines, Maya. *The Brain Changers: Scientists and the New Mind Control.* New York: Harcourt Brace Jovanovich, 1973.

193. Pomeranz, B. "Brain's opiates at work in acupuncture." *New Scientist,* Vol. 6 (1977), pp. 12-13.

194. Ramirez Monzon, Carmenza. "REST and Smoking Cessation in a Latin American Country." Paper delivered at First International Conference on REST and Self-Regulation, Denver, Colorado, March 17, 1983.

195. "Relaxation Tanks: A Market Develops." *The New York Times* (November 21, 1981).

196. Richardson, Alan. *Mental Imagery.* New York: Springer-Verlag, 1969.

197. Rogers, M., D. Dubey, and P. Reich. "The influence of the psyche and the brain on immunity and disease susceptibility: A critical review." *Psychosomatic Medicine,* Vol. 41 (1979), pp. 147-164.

198. Rose, Steven. *The Conscious Brain.* New York: Alfred A. Knopf, 1975.

199. Rosenblatt, Seymour. M.D., and Reynolds Dodson. *Beyond Valium: The Brave New World of Psychochemistry.* New York: G. P. Putnam's Sons, 1981.

200. Rossi, A. M., et al. "Operant Responding for Visual Stimuli during Sensory Deprivation: Effect of Meaningfulness." *Journal of Abnormal Psychology,* Vol. 79 (1969), pp. 188-193.

201. Rossier, J., F. E. Bloom, and R. Guillemin. "Stimulation of human periaqueductal gray for pain relief increases immunoreactive beta-endorphin in ventricular fluid." *Science* (January 19, 1979).

202. Routtenberg, Aryeh. "The Reward System of the Brain." *Scientific American* (November 1978).

203. Russell, Peter. *The Brain Book.* New York: Hawthorn Books, 1979.

204. Sagan, Carl. *Dragons of Eden.* New York: Random House, 1977.

205. Salk, L. "The Role of the Heartbeat in the Relations Between Mother and Infant." *Scientific American* (March 1973).

206. Samuels, Mike, M.D., and Nancy Samuels. *Seeing with the Mind's Eye.* New York: Random House, 1975.

207. Schmeck, Harold M., Jr. "Addict's Brain: Chemistry Holds Hope for Answers." *The New York Times* (January 25, 1983).

208. ————. "The Biology of Fear and Anxiety: Evidence Points to Chemical Triggers." *The New York Times,* (September 7, 1982).

209. ————. "Study Says Smile May Indeed Be an Umbrella." *The New York Times* (September 9, 1983).

210. Schultz. Duane P. *Sensory Restriction: Effects on Behavior.* New York: Academic Press. 1965.

211. Schultz. Johannes. "The clinical importance of 'inward seeing' in autogenic training." *British Journal of Medical Hypnotism,* Vol. 11 (1960). pp. 26-28.

212. ————, and Wolfgang Luthe. *Autogenic Training: A Psychophysiologic Approach in Psychotherapy.* New York: Grune and Stratton. 1959.

213. Scott, Jacque. "Doctors using isolation tank as medical tool." *The Corridor Corral* (November 26, 1981).

214. Selye, Hans. M.D. *The Stress of Life*, rev. ed. New York: McGraw-Hill, 1976.

215. Shafii, Mohammad, M.D., R. Lavely, and R. Jaffe. "Meditation and Marijuana." *American Journal of Psychiatry*, Vol. 131 (1974). pp. 60-63.

216. ———. "Meditation and the Prevention of Drug Abuse." *American Journal of Psychiatry*, Vol. 132 (1975). pp. 942-945.

217. Silverman, Lloyd. "Unconscious Symbiotic Fantasy: A Ubiquitous Therapeutic Agent." *International Journal of Psychoanalytic Psychotherapy*, Vol. 7 (1978-79). p. 568.

218. ———, F. M. Lachmann, and R. H. Milich. *The Search for Oneness.* New York: International Universities Press. 1982.

219. Simonton, O. Carl, Stephanie Matthews-Simonton, and J. Creighton. *Getting Well Again.* Los Angeles: J. P. Tarcher, 1978.

220. ———, and Stephanie Matthews-Simonton. "Belief systems and management of the emotional aspects of malignancy." *Journal of Transpersonal Psychology*, Vol. 7 (197.5). pp. 29-47.

221. Smith, Adam. *Powers of the Mind.* New York: Random House, 1975.

222. Snyder, S. H. "Opiate receptors in the brain." *New England Journal of Medicine* (February 3, 1977).

223. Solomon, Philip. et al., eds. *Sensory Deprivation: A Symposium Held at Harvard Medical School.* Cambridge. Mass.: Harvard University Press. 1961.

224. Sommer. Robert. *The Mind's Eye.* New York: Delacorte Press, 1978.

225. Springer, Sally P.. and Georg Deutsch. *Left Brain. Right Brain.* San Francisco: W. H. Freeman, 1981.

226. Staib, A., and D. N. Logan. "Hypnotic Stimulation of Breast Growth." *American Journal of Clinical Hypnosis*, Vol. 19 (1977). p. 201.

227. Standing. Lionel. "Learning 10,000 Pictures." *Quarterly Journal of Experimental Psychology.* Vol. 25, pp. 207-222.

228. Stanley, John M., William D. Francis, and Heidi Berres. "The Effects of Floatation REST on Cognitive Tasks." Paper delivered at First International Conference on REST and Self-Regulation, Denver, Colorado, March 17. 1983.

229. Stern. Gary S., Ph.D. "Physiological and Mood Effects of Salt Water Floatation Periods." Unpublished paper.

230. Stevens. Charles F. "The Neuron." *Scientific American* (September 1979).

231. "Stress: Can We Cope?" *Time* (June 6, 1983).

232. "Stress Held Factor in I.Q. Scores." *The New York Times* (May 31, 1983).

233. Stuart, Richard B. *Act Thin, Stay Thin.* New York: W. W. Norton. 1978.

234. Suedfeld, Peter. "The Benefits of Boredom: Sensory Deprivation Reconsidered." *American Scientist,* Vol. 63 (1975), pp. 60-69.

235. ———. "The clinical relevance of reduced sensory stimulation." *Canadian Psychological Review,* Vol. 16 (1975). pp. 88-103.

236. ———. "Using environmental restriction to initiate long-term behavioral change." in *Behavioral Self-Management: Strategies, Techniques and Outcomes,* ed. R. B. Stuart. New York: Brunner/Mazel, 1977.

237. ———. *Restricted Environmental Stimulation: Research and Clinical Applications,* New York: John Wiley & Sons. 1980.

238. ———. "REST: Technique. Treatment. Transcendence." Address delivered at First International Conference on REST and Self-Regulation, Denver. Colorado. March 17, 1983.

239. ———, and J. A. Best. "Satiation and sensory deprivation combined in smoking therapy: some case studies and unexpected side-effects. *International Journal of Addiction,* Vol. 12 (1977), pp. 337-359.

240. Suedfeld, Peter. and R. D. Hare. "Sensory deprivation in the treatment of snake phobia: behavioral, self-report and physiological effects." *Behavioral Therapy,* Vol. 8 (1977). pp. 240-50.

241. Suinn, Richard M. "Body Thinking: Psychology for Olympic Champs." *Psychology Today* (July 1976).

242. Szasz, Thomas S.. M.D. *Pain and Pleasure,* 2nd expanded ed. New York: Basic Books, 1975.

243. Tallman, John F., et al. "Receptors for the Age of Anxiety: Pharmacology of the Benzodiazepines." *Science,* Vol. 207 (1980), p. 274.

244. Tart. Charles T., ed. *Altered States of Consciousness.* New York: John Wiley & Sons, 1969.

245. ———. *States of Consciousness.* New York: E. P. Dutton, 1975.

246. Taylor, Gordon Rattray. *The Natural History of the Mind.* New York: E. P. Dutton, 1979.

247. Taylor, Thomas E. "Learning Studies for Higher Cognitive Levels in a Short-term Sensory Isolation Environment." Paper delivered at First International Conference on REST and Self-Regulation, Denver. Colorado. March 17, 1983.

248. ———, Margaret C. Hansen, et al. "A study of EEG as an Indicator of Changes in Cognitive Level of Understanding in a Sensory Isolation Environment." Unpublished paper. Department of Chemistry, Texas A & M University.

249. Tenerowicz, David. "The Tank Center: A Culture Turns Inward." Paper delivered at First International Conference on REST and Self-Regulation, Denver, Colorado. March 17, 1983.

250. Thomas, Lewis, M.D. *The Youngest Science: Notes of a Medicine Watcher.* New York: Viking Press, 1983.

251. Toffler, Alvin. *Previews & Premises.* New York: William Morrow, 1983.

252. Turner, John W. "Hormones and REST: A Controlled Study of REST-Assisted Relaxation." Paper delivered at First International Conference on REST and Self-Regulation, Denver, Colorado, March 18, 1983.

253. "Valium Abuse: The yellow peril." *Time* (September 24, 1979).

254. "Valium Alarm: Does it promote cancer?" *Time* (January 19, 1981).

255. Walford, Roy L., M.D. *Maximum Life Span.* New York: W. W. Norton, 1983.

256. Walkup, Lewis E. "Creativity in Science through Visualization." *Perceptual and Motor Skills,* Vol. 221 (1965), pp. 35-41.

257. Watson, Lyall. *Lifetide: The Biology of the Unconscious.* New York: Simon & Schuster, 1979.

258. Weil, Andrew. *The Natural Mind.* Boston: Houghton Mifflin, 1972.

259. Westcott, M., and J. Ranzoni. "Correlates of Intuitive Thinking." *Psychological Reports,* Vol. 12 (1963), pp. 595-613.

260. Wickramsekera, Ian. "Sensory Restriction and Self-Hypnosis as Potentiators of Self-Regulation." Paper delivered at First International Conference on REST and Self-Regulation, Denver, Colorado, March 18, 1983.

261. Willard, R. D. "Breast Enlargement Through Visual Imagery and Hypnosis." *American Journal of Clinical Hypnosis,* Vol. 19 (1977), p. 195.

262. Williams, J. E. "Stimulation of Breast Growth by Hypnosis." *Journal of Sex Research,* Vol. 10 (1974), pp. 316-324.

263. Witelson, Sandra. "Sex and the Single Hemisphere: Specialization of the Right Hemisphere for Spatial Processing." *Science*, Vol. 193 (1976), pp. 425-426.

264. Wolpe, J. *The Practice of Behavior Therapy.* New York: Pergamon Press, 1969.

265. Woods, Bob. "To Float, Perchance to Dream . . ." *Future Life #25* (March 1981).

266. Woolfolk, Robert L., and Frank C. Richardson. *Stress, Sanity and Survival.* New York: Monarch Press, 1978.

267. Young, J. Z. *Programs of the Brain.* Oxford: Oxford University Press, 1978.

268. Zaidel, Fran. "Unilateral Auditory Language Comprehension on the Token Test Following Cerebral Commissurotomy and Hemispherectomy." *Neuropsychologia* Vol. 15 (1977), pp. 118.

269. Zubek, J. P., ed. *Sensory Deprivation: Fifteen Years of Research.* New York: Appleton-Century-Crofts, 1969.

270. Zuckerman, M. *Sensation Seeking: Beyond the Optimal Level of Arousal.* Hillsdale, N.J.: Lawrence Elbaum Associates, 1979.

Triune brain theory, 65, 69, 155

Ulcers, 48, 93, 97
Ultimate Athlete, The (Leonard), 174
Uncertainty principle, Heisenberg's, 82
Unconscious, the, 91, 135, 140f., 143, 158, 179, 180, 181ff., 212, 222, 226
Unified-field theory of floating, 122
Ursin, Earl, 202

Valium, 205f., 214
Valium receptors, 206
Verbalizers, visualizers versus, 106
Video screens, 169
Videotapes, 222
Visceral brain, 68, 70, 153, 201
Visualization (mental imagery), 7, 59, 72, 103ff., 128, 139, 160ff., 172ff., 199, 207, 214, 218f.
Visuomotor behavior rehearsal technique (VMBR), 174
Walden (Thoreau), 17
Wallace, R. K., 189
Ward, Bob, 170
Water filters, 31
Water heaters, 31
Waters, Charlie, 172
Watson, Lyall, 181
Weight loss, 7, 187, 195ff.
Weight Watchers, 42
Weil, Dr. Andrews 20
Well-being, *see* Health and well-being
Wellness Research Associates, 145
Whirlpool baths, 161
Whitehead, Alfred North, 125
Wickramsekera, Dr. Ian, 49
Williams, Robin, 33
Wilson, Colin, 71
Winter, Bud, 168
Wisdom of the Body, The (Cannon), 121
Withdrawal, 185, 192f.

Dear Reader of *The Book of Floating*,

If you have enjoyed reading this book, and have finally arrived at this last page, you deserve a special reward for your endurance and attention.

This reward comes in the form of a promise. We at Gateways Books and Tapes have now for almost thirty years brought to you the finest spiritual and esoteric classics to you, which are otherwise very hard to find. Our promise is that we will continue to make available to you, our esteemed reader, a selection of the finest consciousness related writings of our times.

For a current catalog and referral to related books and study materials, you may contact Gateways at the address below with no obligation to purchase.

Gateways Books and Tapes
P.O. Box 370-BOF
Nevada City, CA 95959
(800) 869-0658 or (530) 272-0180
www.gatewaysbooksandtapes.com
email: info@gatewaysbooksandtapes.com

A Partial List of Titles You Can Order
(See www.gatewaysbooksandtapes.com for complete current book list)

by Robert S. de Ropp
The Master Game: Pathways to Higher Consciousness
Self-Completion: Keys to a Meaningful Life
Warrior's Way: A Twentieth Century Odyssey

by E.J. Gold
American Book of the Dead
The Great Adventure: Talks on Death, Dying and the Bardos
The Human Biological Machine as a Transformational Apparatus
Practical Work on Self
The Hidden Work
The Seven Bodies of Man
Visions in the Stone: Journey to the Source of Hidden Knowledge
    (Intro. by Robert Anton Wilson)

by John C. Lilly, M.D.
The Deep Self (due in 2004)
with E. J. Gold: *Tanks for the Memories*

by Claudio Naranjo, M.D.
Character & Neurosis: An Integrative View
The Divine Child and the Hero: Inner Meaning in Children's Literature
The Enneagram of Society (due in 2003)

by Reb Zalman Schachter-Shalomi & Howard Schwartz
The Dream Assembly

by Ka-Tzetnik 135633
Shivitti: A Vision

by Dr. Claude Needham, Ph.D.
The Original Handbook for the Recently Deceased

by Mark Olsen
The Golden Buddha Changing Masks: Essays on the Spiritual Dimensions of Acting

For more information about floating and places to float check:
www.floatation.com